Follow this Guide step by step and after 2 months you can be sure to be a normal person with your disturbance under control. It means in 2 months you will not be a person with eating disorder, but a normal one.

Month one

Week One

Day 1

Morning

* Say STOP whenever thoughts about eating come to your mind.

* Say slowly whenever you are invaded by the thoughts about eating: sun, flower, seven, path, tee, run, yellow, apple, fish, rain, pen, water, smile, talk, life, sky.

* If above does not help to stop the thoughts about eating just turn your attention away from the invading thoughts about eating. The best way to turn your attention away from the invading thoughts about eating in your head is by doing one of your favorite occupations. Do not be ashamed of any occupation to turn your attention away from the invading thoughts in your head. ALWAYS be busy with your favorite occupation when unsupportable thoughts come to your head.

* Be careful to keep for yourself these of your believes which are found to be strange by the people.

* CONTROL what you say. Say only things which are not strange for the people. You surely already know which of your believes are found to be strange by the people.

* If you do not know yet which of your believes are found to be strange by the people, OBSERVE how people react on what you say. If you see that people are ALERTED by your believes, it means your believes are strange. From now on AVOID presenting such believes.

* Think of three different words, any words which just come to your mind at the moment and make a simple story using these 3 words. Repeat 3 times.

* Try to concentrate on an object close to you, any object. What do you feel when looking at the object? What thoughts come to your mind when looking at the object? And why?Maybe there is a reason. Look for the reason but not too long. If you don't find the reason, forget it.

* Small physical excercise (10 min)

* Small breakfast.

Can one live, work and be happy with eating disorder (anorexia, boulimia) in a normal way, the way people without eating disorder can? Yes! You can live a normal life with eating disorder. In order to do so there are only 3 steps to do.

First, you should forget eating disorder is a disease, so consequently you are not sick! Of course, you experience some psyche disturbances, but there is no human being on Earth with no disturbance. The number of such disturbances is limitless. But people suffering other disturbances are not considered as sick! Why? It is the question of the history. Some disturbances have become in the 20th century more popularized than others. Since psychiatrists are doctors of medecine they used to call these disturbances „diseases", what is quite easy to understand. But people suffer from limitless number of another different psyche disturbances, which have not become as popular in the 20th century as eating disorders, schizophrenia, depression or anxiety. Believe me, there is no man on Earth without this or that disturbance. Most of us is not treated by psychiatrists because they deal only with the most popular disturbances like: eating disorders, schizophrenia, depression, anxiety. But it does not mean that these are the only disturbances and that these are „diseases". The truth is that there are no diseases in the psychiatry. There are only disturbances.

Second, as the system of the medical care (psychiatrists, hospitals, pharma industry, law, etc) makes permanently sick person out of you, with a label of eating disorder, you have to come back to normal life on your own. But not alone!

Third, you have to be accompanied in your come back to normal life by somobody close to you: a member of your family, friend, anyone you can rely on and someone with no official psychiatric label. It is hard to find such a person, even in the family, because most of the people accept without reflection what doctors (psychiatrists) tell them. They belive in what doctors say and not what you say. But this book can help you to explain it to your family and friends that you are not sick and your desire to live a normal life is fully justified. Remember to show to the people this book. It will open your way to normal life.

In this Guide you will find out how you should proceed step by step, day after day, in order to get rid of this false label of eating disorder, that you are sick. And you will find out how you can overcome your disturbance in order to live a full and normal live.

* Nice talk (no complaints, no problematic questions) 10 min. When nobody to talk with, phone or internet conversation oral or written.

* Walk 15 min.

* If you have invading thoughts about eating, ask yourself if it is possible to ignore them.

Yes

Great! In such a case continue ignoring them.

No

You have to learn to ignore the invading thoughts about eating.

This Guide will teach you to ignore the invading thoughts about eating.

Remember: even if you cannot stop the invading thoughts, the invading thoughts cannot stop you to live a normal life.

If you believe in things which other people consider strange, try to keep your strange believes for yourself. Everybody has to make the selection of what can be told to other people and what must be private. Believe me, many people have strange believes. Even much stranger than yours. And they are not considered to be

sick. Why? Because they keep their strange believes for themselves. That is the secret.

***

Afternoon

* Say slowly whenever you are invaded by the thoughts about eating: sun, flower, seven, path, tee, run, yellow, apple, fish, rain, pen, water, smile, talk, life, sky.

* Think of three different words, any words which just come to your mind at the moment and make a simple story using these 3 words. Repeat 3 times.

* Try to concentrate on an object close to you, any object. What do you feel when looking at the object? What thoughts come to your mind when looking at the object? And why? Maybe there is a reason. Look for the reason but not too long. If you don't find the reason, forget it.

* Dinner and half an hour break (you can sleep).

* Nice talk (no complaints) 15 min. When nobody to talk with, phone or internet conversation oral or written.

* Walk 20 min.

* If you have the invading thoughts about eating, ask yourself if it is possible to ignore them.

Yes

Great! In such a case continue ignoring them.

No

You have to learn to ignore the invading thoughts.

This Guide will teach you to ignore the invading thoughts about eating.

Remember: even if you cannot stop the invading thoughts, the invading thoughts cannot stop you to live a normal life.

If you believe in things which other people consider strange, try to keep your strange believes for yourself. Everybody has to make the selection of what can be told to other people and what must be private. Believe me, many people have strange believes. Even much stranger than yours. And they are not considered to be sick. Why? Because they keep their strange believes for themselves. That is the secret.

***

Evening

- Say slowly whenever you are invaded by the thoughts about eating: sun, flower, seven, path, tee, run, yellow, apple, fish, rain, pen, water, smile, talk, life, sky.

- Think of three different words, any words which just come to your mind at the moment and make a simple story using these 3 words. Repeat 3 times.
  - Try to concentrate on an object close to you, any object. What do you feel when looking at the object? What thoughts come to your mind when looking at the object? And why? Maybe there is a reason. Look for the reason but not too long. If you don't find the reason, forget it.
  - Small supper.
  - Nice talk (no complaints) 10 min. When nobody to talk with, phone or internet conversation oral or written.
  - Walk 10 min.
  - If you have the invading thoughts about eating, ask yourself if it is possible to ignore them.

Yes

Great! In such a case continue ignoring them.

No

You have to learn to ignore the invading thoughts.

This Guide will teach you to ignore the invading thoughts.

Remember: even if you cannot stop the invading thoughts, the invading thoughts cannot stop you to live a normal life.

If you believe in things which other people consider strange, try to keep your strange believes for yourself. Everybody has to make the selection of what can be told to other people and what must be private. Believe me, many people have strange believes. Even much stranger than yours. And they are not considered to be sick. Why? Because they keep their strange believes for themselves. That is the secret.

***

Night

Before sleep

- Take a shower (warm water) 1 min.
- Small physical excercise 3 min.

In Bed

- Repeat STOP (10 times if you have invading thoughts).

- Say slowly whenever you are invaded by the thoughts about eating: sun, flower, seven, path, tee, run, yellow, apple, fish, rain, pen, water, smile, talk, life, sky.
- Think of three different words, any words which just come to your mind at the moment and make a simple story using these 3 words. Repeat untill you fall asleep.

If you cannot fall asleep

- Say slowly whenever you are invaded by the thoughts about eating: sun, flower, seven, path, tee, run, yellow, apple, fish, rain, pen, water, smile, talk, life, sky.

If you cannot asleep

- Think of three different words, any words which just come to your mind at the moment and make a simple story using these 3 words. Repeat untill you fall asleep.

If above does not help

- Stand up and go to the toilet (when possible with as little light as possible)
- Say slowly whenever you are invaded by the thoughts about eating: sun, flower, seven, path,

tee, run, yellow, apple, fish, rain, pen, water, smile, talk, life, sky.
- Think of three different words, any words which just come to your mind at the moment and make a simple story using these 3 words. Repeat untill you fall asleep.

If above does not help
- Say STOP untill you fall asleep

If above does not help
- Go to the kitchen and have a very small snack.
- Back to the bed think of three different words, any words which just come to your mind at the moment and make a simple story using these 3 words. Repeat untill you fall asleep.
- If above does not help think of three different words, any words which just come to your mind at the moment and make a simple story using these 3 words. Repeat untill you fall asleep.
- Say slowly whenever you are invaded by the thoughts about eating: sun, flower, seven, path, tee, run, yellow, apple, fish, rain, pen, water, smile, talk, life, sky. Repeat untill you fall asleep.

***

Day 2

Morning

* Say STOP whenever thoughts about eating come to your mind.

* Say slowly whenever you are invaded by the thoughts about eating: sun, flower, seven, path, tee, run, yellow, apple, fish, rain, pen, water, smile, talk, life, sky.

* If above does not help to stop the thoughts about eating just turn your attention away from the invading thoughts about eating. The best way to turn your attention away from the invading thoughts about eating in your head is by doing one of your favorite occupations. Do not be ashamed of any occupation to turn your attention away from the invading thoughts in your head. ALWAYS be busy with your favorite occupation when unsupportable thoughts come to your head.

* Be careful to keep for yourself these of your believes which are found to be strange by the people.

* CONTROL what you say. Say only things which are not strange for the people. You surely already know which of your believes are found to be strange by the people.

* If you do not know yet which of your believes are found to be strange by the people, OBSERVE how

people react on what you say. If you see that people are ALERTED by your believes, it means your believes are strange. From now on AVOID presenting such believes.

* Think of three different words, any words which just come to your mind at the moment and make a simple story using these 3 words. Repeat 3 times.

* Try to concentrate on an object close to you, any object. What do you feel when looking at the object? What thoughts come to your mind when looking at the object? And why? Maybe there is a reason. Look for the reason but not too long. If you don't find the reason, forget it.

* Small physical excercise (10 min)

* Small breakfast.

* Nice talk (no complaints, no problematic questions) 10 min. When nobody to talk with, phone or internet conversation oral or written.

* Walk 15 min.

* If you have invading thoughts about eating, ask yourself if it is possible to ignore them.

Yes

Great! In such a case continue ignoring them.

No

You have to learn to ignore the invading thoughts about eating.

This Guide will teach you to ignore the invading thoughts about eating.

Remember: even if you cannot stop the invading thoughts, the invading thoughts cannot stop you to live a normal life.

If you believe in things which other people consider strange, try to keep your strange believes for yourself. Everybody has to make the selection of what can be told to other people and what must be private. Believe me, many people have strange believes. Even much stranger than yours. And they are not considered to be sick. Why? Because they keep their strange believes for themselves. That is the secret.

***

Afternoon

* Say slowly whenever you are invaded by the thoughts about eating: sun, flower, seven, path, tee, run, yellow, apple, fish, rain, pen, water, smile, talk, life, sky.

* Think of three different words, any words which just come to your mind at the moment and make a simple story using these 3 words. Repeat 3 times.

* Try to concentrate on an object close to you, any object. What do you feel when looking at the object? What thoughts come to your mind when looking at the object? And why?Maybe there is a reason. Look for the reason but not too long. If you don't find the reason, forget it.

* Dinner and half an hour break (you can sleep).

* Nice talk (no complaints) 15 min. When nobody to talk with, phone or internet conversation oral or written.

* Walk 20 min.

* If you have the invading thoughts about eating, ask yourself if it is possible to ignore them.

Yes

Great! In such a case continue ignoring them.

No

You have to learn to ignore the invading thoughts.

This Guide will teach you to ignore the invading thoughts about eating.

Remember: even if you cannot stop the invading thoughts, the invading thoughts cannot stop you to live a normal life.

If you believe in things which other people consider strange, try to keep your strange believes for yourself. Everybody has to make the selection of what can be told to other people and what must be private. Believe me, many people have strange believes. Even much stranger than yours. And they are not considered to be sick. Why? Because they keep their strange believes for themselves. That is the secret.

***

Evening

- Say slowly whenever you are invaded by the thoughts about eating: sun, flower, seven, path, tee, run, yellow, apple, fish, rain, pen, water, smile, talk, life, sky.

- Think of three different words, any words which just come to your mind at the moment and make a simple story using these 3 words. Repeat 3 times.
  - Try to concentrate on an object close to you, any object. What do you feel when looking at the object? What thoughts come to your mind when

looking at the object? And why? Maybe there is a reason. Look for the reason but not too long. If you don't find the reason, forget it.
- Small supper.
- Nice talk (no complaints) 10 min. When nobody to talk with, phone or internet conversation oral or written.
- Walk 10 min.
- If you have the invading thoughts about eating, ask yourself if it is possible to ignore them.

Yes

Great! In such a case continue ignoring them.

No

You have to learn to ignore the invading thoughts.

This Guide will teach you to ignore the invading thoughts.

Remember: even if you cannot stop the invading thoughts, the invading thoughts cannot stop you to live a normal life.

If you believe in things which other people consider strange, try to keep your strange believes for yourself. Everybody has to make the selection of what can be told to other people and what must be private. Believe

me, many people have strange believes. Even much stranger than yours. And they are not considered to be sick. Why? Because they keep their strange believes for themselves. That is the secret.

***

Night

Before sleep

- Take a shower (warm water) 1 min.
- Small physical excercise 3 min.

In Bed

- Repeat STOP (10 times if you have invading thoughts).
- Say slowly whenever you are invaded by the thoughts about eating: sun, flower, seven, path, tee, run, yellow, apple, fish, rain, pen, water, smile, talk, life, sky.
- Think of three different words, any words which just come to your mind at the moment and make a simple story using these 3 words. Repeat untill you fall asleep.

If you cannot fall asleep

- Say slowly whenever you are invaded by the thoughts about eating: sun, flower, seven, path,

tee, run, yellow, apple, fish, rain, pen, water, smile, talk, life, sky.

If you cannot asleep

- Think of three different words, any words which just come to your mind at the moment and make a simple story using these 3 words. Repeat untill you fall asleep.

If above does not help

- Stand up and go to the toilet (when possible with as little light as possible)
- Say slowly whenever you are invaded by the thoughts about eating: sun, flower, seven, path, tee, run, yellow, apple, fish, rain, pen, water, smile, talk, life, sky.
- Think of three different words, any words which just come to your mind at the moment and make a simple story using these 3 words. Repeat untill you fall asleep.

If above does not help

- Say STOP untill you fall asleep

If above does not help

- Go to the kitchen and have a very small snack.

- Back to the bed think of three different words, any words which just come to your mind at the moment and make a simple story using these 3 words. Repeat untill you fall asleep.
- If above does not help think of three different words, any words which just come to your mind at the moment and make a simple story using these 3 words. Repeat untill you fall asleep.
- Say slowly whenever you are invaded by the thoughts about eating: sun, flower, seven, path, tee, run, yellow, apple, fish, rain, pen, water, smile, talk, life, sky. Repeat untill you fall asleep.

***

Day 3

Morning

* Say STOP whenever thoughts about eating come to your mind.

* Say slowly whenever you are invaded by the thoughts about eating: sun, flower, seven, path, tee, run, yellow, apple, fish, rain, pen, water, smile, talk, life, sky.

* If above does not help to stop the thoughts about eating just turn your attention away from the invading thoughts about eating. The best way to turn your

attention away from the invading thoughts about eating in your head is by doing one of your favorite occupations. Do not be ashamed of any occupation to turn your attention away from the invading thoughts in your head. ALWAYS be busy with your favorite occupation when unsupportable thoughts come to your head.

* Be careful to keep for yourself these of your believes which are found to be strange by the people.

* CONTROL what you say. Say only things which are not strange for the people. You surely already know which of your believes are found to be strange by the people.

* If you do not know yet which of your believes are found to be strange by the people, OBSERVE how people react on what you say. If you see that people are ALERTED by your believes, it means your believes are strange. From now on AVOID presenting such believes.

* Think of three different words, any words which just come to your mind at the moment and make a simple story using these 3 words. Repeat 3 times.

* Try to concentrate on an object close to you, any object. What do you feel when looking at the object? What thoughts come to your mind when looking at the object? And why? Maybe there is a reason. Look for the

reason but not too long. If you don't find the reason, forget it.

* Small physical excercise (10 min)

* Small breakfast.

* Nice talk (no complaints, no problematic questions) 10 min. When nobody to talk with, phone or internet conversation oral or written.

* Walk 15 min.

* If you have invading thoughts about eating, ask yourself if it is possible to ignore them.

Yes

Great! In such a case continue ignoring them.

No

You have to learn to ignore the invading thoughts about eating.

This Guide will teach you to ignore the invading thoughts about eating.

Remember: even if you cannot stop the invading thoughts, the invading thoughts cannot stop you to live a normal life.

If you believe in things which other people consider strange, try to keep your strange believes for yourself. Everybody has to make the selection of what can be told to other people and what must be private. Believe me, many people have strange believes. Even much stranger than yours. And they are not considered to be sick. Why? Because they keep their strange believes for themselves. That is the secret.

***

Afternoon

* Say slowly whenever you are invaded by the thoughts about eating: sun, flower, seven, path, tee, run, yellow, apple, fish, rain, pen, water, smile, talk, life, sky.

* Think of three different words, any words which just come to your mind at the moment and make a simple story using these 3 words. Repeat 3 times.

* Try to concentrate on an object close to you, any object. What do you feel when looking at the object? What thoughts come to your mind when looking at the object? And why? Maybe there is a reason. Look for the reason but not too long. If you don't find the reason, forget it.

* Dinner and half an hour break (you can sleep).

* Nice talk (no complaints) 15 min. When nobody to talk with, phone or internet conversation oral or written.

* Walk 20 min.

* If you have the invading thoughts about eating, ask yourself if it is possible to ignore them.

Yes

Great! In such a case continue ignoring them.

No

You have to learn to ignore the invading thoughts.

This Guide will teach you to ignore the invading thoughts about eating.

Remember: even if you cannot stop the invading thoughts, the invading thoughts cannot stop you to live a normal life.

If you believe in things which other people consider strange, try to keep your strange believes for yourself. Everybody has to make the selection of what can be told to other people and what must be private. Believe me, many people have strange believes. Even much stranger than yours. And they are not considered to be

sick. Why? Because they keep their strange believes for themselves. That is the secret.

***

Evening

- Say slowly whenever you are invaded by the thoughts about eating: sun, flower, seven, path, tee, run, yellow, apple, fish, rain, pen, water, smile, talk, life, sky.

- Think of three different words, any words which just come to your mind at the moment and make a simple story using these 3 words. Repeat 3 times.
  - Try to concentrate on an object close to you, any object. What do you feel when looking at the object? What thoughts come to your mind when looking at the object? And why? Maybe there is a reason. Look for the reason but not too long. If you don't find the reason, forget it.
  - Small supper.
  - Nice talk (no complaints) 10 min. When nobody to talk with, phone or internet conversation oral or written.
  - Walk 10 min.
  - If you have the invading thoughts about eating, ask yourself if it is possible to ignore them.

Yes

Great! In such a case continue ignoring them.

No

You have to learn to ignore the invading thoughts.

This Guide will teach you to ignore the invading thoughts.

Remember: even if you cannot stop the invading thoughts, the invading thoughts cannot stop you to live a normal life.

If you believe in things which other people consider strange, try to keep your strange believes for yourself. Everybody has to make the selection of what can be told to other people and what must be private. Believe me, many people have strange believes. Even much stranger than yours. And they are not considered to be sick. Why? Because they keep their strange believes for themselves. That is the secret.

***

Night

Before sleep

- Take a shower (warm water) 1 min.
- Small physical excercise 3 min.

In Bed

- Repeat STOP (10 times if you have invading thoughts).
- Say slowly whenever you are invaded by the thoughts about eating: sun, flower, seven, path, tee, run, yellow, apple, fish, rain, pen, water, smile, talk, life, sky.
- Think of three different words, any words which just come to your mind at the moment and make a simple story using these 3 words. Repeat untill you fall asleep.

If you cannot fall asleep

- Say slowly whenever you are invaded by the thoughts about eating: sun, flower, seven, path, tee, run, yellow, apple, fish, rain, pen, water, smile, talk, life, sky.

If you cannot asleep

- Think of three different words, any words which just come to your mind at the moment and make a simple story using these 3 words. Repeat untill you fall asleep.

If above does not help

- Stand up and go to the toilet (when possible with as little light as possible)

- Say slowly whenever you are invaded by the thoughts about eating: sun, flower, seven, path, tee, run, yellow, apple, fish, rain, pen, water, smile, talk, life, sky.
- Think of three different words, any words which just come to your mind at the moment and make a simple story using these 3 words. Repeat untill you fall asleep.

If above does not help

- Say STOP untill you fall asleep

If above does not help

- Go to the kitchen and have a very small snack.
- Back to the bed think of three different words, any words which just come to your mind at the moment and make a simple story using these 3 words. Repeat untill you fall asleep.
- If above does not help think of three different words, any words which just come to your mind at the moment and make a simple story using these 3 words. Repeat untill you fall asleep.
- Say slowly whenever you are invaded by the thoughts about eating: sun, flower, seven, path, tee, run, yellow, apple, fish, rain, pen, water, smile, talk, life, sky. Repeat untill you fall asleep.

***

Day 4

Morning

* Say STOP whenever thoughts about eating come to your mind.

* Say slowly whenever you are invaded by the thoughts about eating: sun, flower, seven, path, tee, run, yellow, apple, fish, rain, pen, water, smile, talk, life, sky.

* If above does not help to stop the thoughts about eating just turn your attention away from the invading thoughts about eating. The best way to turn your attention away from the invading thoughts about eating in your head is by doing one of your favorite occupations. Do not be ashamed of any occupation to turn your attention away from the invading thoughts in your head. ALWAYS be busy with your favorite occupation when unsupportable thoughts come to your head.

* Be careful to keep for yourself these of your believes which are found to be strange by the people.

* CONTROL what you say. Say only things which are not strange for the people. You surely already know which of your believes are found to be strange by the people.

* If you do not know yet which of your believes are found to be strange by the people, OBSERVE how people react on what you say. If you see that people are ALERTED by your believes, it means your believes are strange. From now on AVOID presenting such believes.

* Think of three different words, any words which just come to your mind at the moment and make a simple story using these 3 words. Repeat 3 times.

* Try to concentrate on an object close to you, any object. What do you feel when looking at the object? What thoughts come to your mind when looking at the object? And why? Maybe there is a reason. Look for the reason but not too long. If you don't find the reason, forget it.

* Small physical excercise (10 min)

* Small breakfast.

* Nice talk (no complaints, no problematic questions) 10 min. When nobody to talk with, phone or internet conversation oral or written.

* Walk 15 min.

* If you have invading thoughts about eating, ask yourself if it is possible to ignore them.

Yes

Great! In such a case continue ignoring them.

No

You have to learn to ignore the invading thoughts about eating.

This Guide will teach you to ignore the invading thoughts about eating.

Remember: even if you cannot stop the invading thoughts, the invading thoughts cannot stop you to live a normal life.

If you believe in things which other people consider strange, try to keep your strange believes for yourself. Everybody has to make the selection of what can be told to other people and what must be private. Believe me, many people have strange believes. Even much stranger than yours. And they are not considered to be sick. Why? Because they keep their strange believes for themselves. That is the secret.

***

Afternoon

* Say slowly whenever you are invaded by the thoughts about eating: sun, flower, seven, path, tee, run, yellow, apple, fish, rain, pen, water, smile, talk, life, sky.

* Think of three different words, any words which just come to your mind at the moment and make a simple story using these 3 words. Repeat 3 times.

* Try to concentrate on an object close to you, any object. What do you feel when looking at the object? What thoughts come to your mind when looking at the object? And why? Maybe there is a reason. Look for the reason but not too long. If you don't find the reason, forget it.

* Dinner and half an hour break (you can sleep).

* Nice talk (no complaints) 15 min. When nobody to talk with, phone or internet conversation oral or written.

* Walk 20 min.

* If you have the invading thoughts about eating, ask yourself if it is possible to ignore them.

Yes

Great! In such a case continue ignoring them.

No

You have to learn to ignore the invading thoughts.

This Guide will teach you to ignore the invading thoughts about eating.

Remember: even if you cannot stop the invading thoughts, the invading thoughts cannot stop you to live a normal life.

If you believe in things which other people consider strange, try to keep your strange believes for yourself. Everybody has to make the selection of what can be told to other people and what must be private. Believe me, many people have strange believes. Even much stranger than yours. And they are not considered to be sick. Why? Because they keep their strange believes for themselves. That is the secret.

***

Evening

- Say slowly whenever you are invaded by the thoughts about eating: sun, flower, seven, path, tee, run, yellow, apple, fish, rain, pen, water, smile, talk, life, sky.

- Think of three different words, any words which just come to your mind at the moment and make a simple story using these 3 words. Repeat 3 times.

- Try to concentrate on an object close to you, any object. What do you feel when looking at the object? What thoughts come to your mind when looking at the object? And why? Maybe there is a reason. Look for the reason but not too long. If you don't find the reason, forget it.
- Small supper.
- Nice talk (no complaints) 10 min. When nobody to talk with, phone or internet conversation oral or written.
- Walk 10 min.
- If you have the invading thoughts about eating, ask yourself if it is possible to ignore them.

Yes

Great! In such a case continue ignoring them.

No

You have to learn to ignore the invading thoughts.

This Guide will teach you to ignore the invading thoughts.

Remember: even if you cannot stop the invading thoughts, the invading thoughts cannot stop you to live a normal life.

If you believe in things which other people consider strange, try to keep your strange believes for yourself. Everybody has to make the selection of what can be told to other people and what must be private. Believe me, many people have strange believes. Even much stranger than yours. And they are not considered to be sick. Why? Because they keep their strange believes for themselves. That is the secret.

***

Night

Before sleep

- Take a shower (warm water) 1 min.
- Small physical excercise 3 min.

In Bed

- Repeat STOP (10 times if you have invading thoughts).
- Say slowly whenever you are invaded by the thoughts about eating: sun, flower, seven, path, tee, run, yellow, apple, fish, rain, pen, water, smile, talk, life, sky.
- Think of three different words, any words which just come to your mind at the moment and make a simple story using these 3 words. Repeat untill you fall asleep.

If you cannot fall asleep

- Say slowly whenever you are invaded by the thoughts about eating: sun, flower, seven, path, tee, run, yellow, apple, fish, rain, pen, water, smile, talk, life, sky.

If you cannot asleep

- Think of three different words, any words which just come to your mind at the moment and make a simple story using these 3 words. Repeat untill you fall asleep.

If above does not help

- Stand up and go to the toilet (when possible with as little light as possible)
- Say slowly whenever you are invaded by the thoughts about eating: sun, flower, seven, path, tee, run, yellow, apple, fish, rain, pen, water, smile, talk, life, sky.
- Think of three different words, any words which just come to your mind at the moment and make a simple story using these 3 words. Repeat untill you fall asleep.

If above does not help

- Say STOP untill you fall asleep

If above does not help

- Go to the kitchen and have a very small snack.
- Back to the bed think of three different words, any words which just come to your mind at the moment and make a simple story using these 3 words. Repeat untill you fall asleep.
- If above does not help think of three different words, any words which just come to your mind at the moment and make a simple story using these 3 words. Repeat untill you fall asleep.
- Say slowly whenever you are invaded by the thoughts about eating: sun, flower, seven, path, tee, run, yellow, apple, fish, rain, pen, water, smile, talk, life, sky. Repeat untill you fall asleep.

***

Day 5

Morning

* Say STOP whenever thoughts about eating come to your mind.

* Say slowly whenever you are invaded by the thoughts about eating: sun, flower, seven, path, tee, run, yellow, apple, fish, rain, pen, water, smile, talk, life, sky.

* If above does not help to stop the thoughts about eating just turn your attention away from the invading thoughts about eating. The best way to turn your attention away from the invading thoughts about eating in your head is by doing one of your favorite occupations. Do not be ashamed of any occupation to turn your attention away from the invading thoughts in your head. ALWAYS be busy with your favorite occupation when unsupportable thoughts come to your head.

* Be careful to keep for yourself these of your believes which are found to be strange by the people.

* CONTROL what you say. Say only things which are not strange for the people. You surely already know which of your believes are found to be strange by the people.

* If you do not know yet which of your believes are found to be strange by the people, OBSERVE how people react on what you say. If you see that people are ALERTED by your believes, it means your believes are strange. From now on AVOID presenting such believes.

* Think of three different words, any words which just come to your mind at the moment and make a simple story using these 3 words. Repeat 3 times.

* Try to concentrate on an object close to you, any object. What do you feel when looking at the object? What thoughts come to your mind when looking at the object? And why?Maybe there is a reason. Look for the reason but not too long. If you don't find the reason, forget it.

* Small physical excercise (10 min)

* Small breakfast.

* Nice talk (no complaints, no problematic questions) 10 min. When nobody to talk with, phone or internet conversation oral or written.

* Walk 15 min.

* If you have invading thoughts about eating, ask yourself if it is possible to ignore them.

Yes

Great! In such a case continue ignoring them.

No

You have to learn to ignore the invading thoughts about eating.

This Guide will teach you to ignore the invading thoughts about eating.

Remember: even if you cannot stop the invading thoughts, the invading thoughts cannot stop you to live a normal life.

If you believe in things which other people consider strange, try to keep your strange believes for yourself. Everybody has to make the selection of what can be told to other people and what must be private. Believe me, many people have strange believes. Even much stranger than yours. And they are not considered to be sick. Why? Because they keep their strange believes for themselves. That is the secret.

***

Afternoon

* Say slowly whenever you are invaded by the thoughts about eating: sun, flower, seven, path, tee, run, yellow, apple, fish, rain, pen, water, smile, talk, life, sky.

* Think of three different words, any words which just come to your mind at the moment and make a simple story using these 3 words. Repeat 3 times.

* Try to concentrate on an object close to you, any object. What do you feel when looking at the object? What thoughts come to your mind when looking at the

object? And why? Maybe there is a reason. Look for the reason but not too long. If you don't find the reason, forget it.

* Dinner and half an hour break (you can sleep).

* Nice talk (no complaints) 15 min. When nobody to talk with, phone or internet conversation oral or written.

* Walk 20 min.

* If you have the invading thoughts about eating, ask yourself if it is possible to ignore them.

Yes

Great! In such a case continue ignoring them.

No

You have to learn to ignore the invading thoughts.

This Guide will teach you to ignore the invading thoughts about eating.

Remember: even if you cannot stop the invading thoughts, the invading thoughts cannot stop you to live a normal life.

If you believe in things which other people consider strange, try to keep your strange believes for yourself. Everybody has to make the selection of what can be

told to other people and what must be private. Believe me, many people have strange believes. Even much stranger than yours. And they are not considered to be sick. Why? Because they keep their strange believes for themselves. That is the secret.

***

Evening

- Say slowly whenever you are invaded by the thoughts about eating: sun, flower, seven, path, tee, run, yellow, apple, fish, rain, pen, water, smile, talk, life, sky.

- Think of three different words, any words which just come to your mind at the moment and make a simple story using these 3 words. Repeat 3 times.
  - Try to concentrate on an object close to you, any object. What do you feel when looking at the object? What thoughts come to your mind when looking at the object? And why?Maybe there is a reason. Look for the reason but not too long. If you don't find the reason, forget it.
  - Small supper.
  - Nice talk (no complaints) 10 min. When nobody to talk with, phone or internet conversation oral or written.

- Walk 10 min.
- If you have the invading thoughts about eating, ask yourself if it is possible to ignore them.

Yes

Great! In such a case continue ignoring them.

No

You have to learn to ignore the invading thoughts.

This Guide will teach you to ignore the invading thoughts.

Remember: even if you cannot stop the invading thoughts, the invading thoughts cannot stop you to live a normal life.

If you believe in things which other people consider strange, try to keep your strange believes for yourself. Everybody has to make the selection of what can be told to other people and what must be private. Believe me, many people have strange believes. Even much stranger than yours. And they are not considered to be sick. Why? Because they keep their strange believes for themselves. That is the secret.

***

Night

Before sleep

- Take a shower (warm water) 1 min.
- Small physical excercise 3 min.

In Bed

- Repeat STOP (10 times if you have invading thoughts).
- Say slowly whenever you are invaded by the thoughts about eating: sun, flower, seven, path, tee, run, yellow, apple, fish, rain, pen, water, smile, talk, life, sky.
- Think of three different words, any words which just come to your mind at the moment and make a simple story using these 3 words. Repeat untill you fall asleep.

If you cannot fall asleep

- Say slowly whenever you are invaded by the thoughts about eating: sun, flower, seven, path, tee, run, yellow, apple, fish, rain, pen, water, smile, talk, life, sky.

If you cannot asleep

- Think of three different words, any words which just come to your mind at the moment and make a simple story using these 3 words. Repeat untill you fall asleep.

If above does not help

- Stand up and go to the toilet (when possible with as little light as possible)
- Say slowly whenever you are invaded by the thoughts about eating: sun, flower, seven, path, tee, run, yellow, apple, fish, rain, pen, water, smile, talk, life, sky.
- Think of three different words, any words which just come to your mind at the moment and make a simple story using these 3 words. Repeat untill you fall asleep.

If above does not help

- Say STOP untill you fall asleep

If above does not help

- Go to the kitchen and have a very small snack.
- Back to the bed think of three different words, any words which just come to your mind at the moment and make a simple story using these 3 words. Repeat untill you fall asleep.
- If above does not help think of three different words, any words which just come to your mind at the moment and make a simple story using these 3 words. Repeat untill you fall asleep.

- Say slowly whenever you are invaded by the thoughts about eating: sun, flower, seven, path, tee, run, yellow, apple, fish, rain, pen, water, smile, talk, life, sky. Repeat untill you fall asleep.

***

Day 6

Morning

* Say STOP whenever thoughts about eating come to your mind.

* Say slowly whenever you are invaded by the thoughts about eating: sun, flower, seven, path, tee, run, yellow, apple, fish, rain, pen, water, smile, talk, life, sky.

* If above does not help to stop the thoughts about eating just turn your attention away from the invading thoughts about eating. The best way to turn your attention away from the invading thoughts about eating in your head is by doing one of your favorite occupations. Do not be ashamed of any occupation to turn your attention away from the invading thoughts in your head. ALWAYS be busy with your favorite occupation when unsupportable thoughts come to your head.

* Be careful to keep for yourself these of your believes which are found to be strange by the people.

* CONTROL what you say. Say only things which are not strange for the people. You surely already know which of your believes are found to be strange by the people.

* If you do not know yet which of your believes are found to be strange by the people, OBSERVE how people react on what you say. If you see that people are ALERTED by your believes, it means your believes are strange. From now on AVOID presenting such believes.

* Think of three different words, any words which just come to your mind at the moment and make a simple story using these 3 words. Repeat 3 times.

* Try to concentrate on an object close to you, any object. What do you feel when looking at the object? What thoughts come to your mind when looking at the object? And why?Maybe there is a reason. Look for the reason but not too long. If you don't find the reason, forget it.

* Small physical excercise (10 min)

* Small breakfast.

* Nice talk (no complaints, no problematic questions) 10 min. When nobody to talk with, phone or internet conversation oral or written.

* Walk 15 min.

* If you have invading thoughts about eating, ask yourself if it is possible to ignore them.

Yes

Great! In such a case continue ignoring them.

No

You have to learn to ignore the invading thoughts about eating.

This Guide will teach you to ignore the invading thoughts about eating.

Remember: even if you cannot stop the invading thoughts, the invading thoughts cannot stop you to live a normal life.

If you believe in things which other people consider strange, try to keep your strange believes for yourself. Everybody has to make the selection of what can be told to other people and what must be private. Believe me, many people have strange believes. Even much stranger than yours. And they are not considered to be

sick. Why? Because they keep their strange believes for themselves. That is the secret.

***

Afternoon

* Say slowly whenever you are invaded by the thoughts about eating: sun, flower, seven, path, tee, run, yellow, apple, fish, rain, pen, water, smile, talk, life, sky.

* Think of three different words, any words which just come to your mind at the moment and make a simple story using these 3 words. Repeat 3 times.

* Try to concentrate on an object close to you, any object. What do you feel when looking at the object? What thoughts come to your mind when looking at the object? And why? Maybe there is a reason. Look for the reason but not too long. If you don't find the reason, forget it.

* Dinner and half an hour break (you can sleep).

* Nice talk (no complaints) 15 min. When nobody to talk with, phone or internet conversation oral or written.

* Walk 20 min.

* If you have the invading thoughts about eating, ask yourself if it is possible to ignore them.

Yes

Great! In such a case continue ignoring them.

No

You have to learn to ignore the invading thoughts.

This Guide will teach you to ignore the invading thoughts about eating.

Remember: even if you cannot stop the invading thoughts, the invading thoughts cannot stop you to live a normal life.

If you believe in things which other people consider strange, try to keep your strange believes for yourself. Everybody has to make the selection of what can be told to other people and what must be private. Believe me, many people have strange believes. Even much stranger than yours. And they are not considered to be sick. Why? Because they keep their strange believes for themselves. That is the secret.

***

Evening

- Say slowly whenever you are invaded by the thoughts about eating: sun, flower, seven, path, tee, run, yellow, apple, fish, rain, pen, water, smile, talk, life, sky.

- Think of three different words, any words which just come to your mind at the moment and make a simple story using these 3 words. Repeat 3 times.
  - Try to concentrate on an object close to you, any object. What do you feel when looking at the object? What thoughts come to your mind when looking at the object? And why? Maybe there is a reason. Look for the reason but not too long. If you don't find the reason, forget it.
  - Small supper.
  - Nice talk (no complaints) 10 min. When nobody to talk with, phone or internet conversation oral or written.
  - Walk 10 min.
  - If you have the invading thoughts about eating, ask yourself if it is possible to ignore them.

Yes

Great! In such a case continue ignoring them.

No

You have to learn to ignore the invading thoughts.

This Guide will teach you to ignore the invading thoughts.

Remember: even if you cannot stop the invading thoughts, the invading thoughts cannot stop you to live a normal life.

If you believe in things which other people consider strange, try to keep your strange believes for yourself. Everybody has to make the selection of what can be told to other people and what must be private. Believe me, many people have strange believes. Even much stranger than yours. And they are not considered to be sick. Why? Because they keep their strange believes for themselves. That is the secret.

***

Night

Before sleep

- Take a shower (warm water) 1 min.
- Small physical excercise 3 min.

In Bed

- Repeat STOP (10 times if you have invading thoughts).

- Say slowly whenever you are invaded by the thoughts about eating: sun, flower, seven, path, tee, run, yellow, apple, fish, rain, pen, water, smile, talk, life, sky.
- Think of three different words, any words which just come to your mind at the moment and make a simple story using these 3 words. Repeat untill you fall asleep.

If you cannot fall asleep

- Say slowly whenever you are invaded by the thoughts about eating: sun, flower, seven, path, tee, run, yellow, apple, fish, rain, pen, water, smile, talk, life, sky.

If you cannot asleep

- Think of three different words, any words which just come to your mind at the moment and make a simple story using these 3 words. Repeat untill you fall asleep.

If above does not help

- Stand up and go to the toilet (when possible with as little light as possible)
- Say slowly whenever you are invaded by the thoughts about eating: sun, flower, seven, path,

tee, run, yellow, apple, fish, rain, pen, water, smile, talk, life, sky.
- Think of three different words, any words which just come to your mind at the moment and make a simple story using these 3 words. Repeat untill you fall asleep.

If above does not help

- Say STOP untill you fall asleep

If above does not help

- Go to the kitchen and have a very small snack.
- Back to the bed think of three different words, any words which just come to your mind at the moment and make a simple story using these 3 words. Repeat untill you fall asleep.
- If above does not help think of three different words, any words which just come to your mind at the moment and make a simple story using these 3 words. Repeat untill you fall asleep.
- Say slowly whenever you are invaded by the thoughts about eating: sun, flower, seven, path, tee, run, yellow, apple, fish, rain, pen, water, smile, talk, life, sky. Repeat untill you fall asleep.

***

Day 7

Morning

* Say STOP whenever thoughts about eating come to your mind.

* Say slowly whenever you are invaded by the thoughts about eating: sun, flower, seven, path, tee, run, yellow, apple, fish, rain, pen, water, smile, talk, life, sky.

* If above does not help to stop the thoughts about eating just turn your attention away from the invading thoughts about eating. The best way to turn your attention away from the invading thoughts about eating in your head is by doing one of your favorite occupations. Do not be ashamed of any occupation to turn your attention away from the invading thoughts in your head. ALWAYS be busy with your favorite occupation when unsupportable thoughts come to your head.

* Be careful to keep for yourself these of your believes which are found to be strange by the people.

* CONTROL what you say. Say only things which are not strange for the people. You surely already know which of your believes are found to be strange by the people.

* If you do not know yet which of your believes are found to be strange by the people, OBSERVE how

people react on what you say. If you see that people are ALERTED by your believes, it means your believes are strange. From now on AVOID presenting such believes.

* Think of three different words, any words which just come to your mind at the moment and make a simple story using these 3 words. Repeat 3 times.

* Try to concentrate on an object close to you, any object. What do you feel when looking at the object? What thoughts come to your mind when looking at the object? And why? Maybe there is a reason. Look for the reason but not too long. If you don't find the reason, forget it.

* Small physical excercise (10 min)

* Small breakfast.

* Nice talk (no complaints, no problematic questions) 10 min. When nobody to talk with, phone or internet conversation oral or written.

* Walk 15 min.

* If you have invading thoughts about eating, ask yourself if it is possible to ignore them.

Yes

Great! In such a case continue ignoring them.

No

You have to learn to ignore the invading thoughts about eating.

This Guide will teach you to ignore the invading thoughts about eating.

Remember: even if you cannot stop the invading thoughts, the invading thoughts cannot stop you to live a normal life.

If you believe in things which other people consider strange, try to keep your strange believes for yourself. Everybody has to make the selection of what can be told to other people and what must be private. Believe me, many people have strange believes. Even much stranger than yours. And they are not considered to be sick. Why? Because they keep their strange believes for themselves. That is the secret.

***

Afternoon

* Say slowly whenever you are invaded by the thoughts about eating: sun, flower, seven, path, tee, run, yellow, apple, fish, rain, pen, water, smile, talk, life, sky.

* Think of three different words, any words which just come to your mind at the moment and make a simple story using these 3 words. Repeat 3 times.

* Try to concentrate on an object close to you, any object. What do you feel when looking at the object? What thoughts come to your mind when looking at the object? And why? Maybe there is a reason. Look for the reason but not too long. If you don't find the reason, forget it.

* Dinner and half an hour break (you can sleep).

* Nice talk (no complaints) 15 min. When nobody to talk with, phone or internet conversation oral or written.

* Walk 20 min.

* If you have the invading thoughts about eating, ask yourself if it is possible to ignore them.

Yes

Great! In such a case continue ignoring them.

No

You have to learn to ignore the invading thoughts.

This Guide will teach you to ignore the invading thoughts about eating.

Remember: even if you cannot stop the invading thoughts, the invading thoughts cannot stop you to live a normal life.

If you believe in things which other people consider strange, try to keep your strange believes for yourself. Everybody has to make the selection of what can be told to other people and what must be private. Believe me, many people have strange believes. Even much stranger than yours. And they are not considered to be sick. Why? Because they keep their strange believes for themselves. That is the secret.

***

Evening

- Say slowly whenever you are invaded by the thoughts about eating: sun, flower, seven, path, tee, run, yellow, apple, fish, rain, pen, water, smile, talk, life, sky.

- Think of three different words, any words which just come to your mind at the moment and make a simple story using these 3 words. Repeat 3 times.
    - Try to concentrate on an object close to you, any object. What do you feel when looking at the object? What thoughts come to your mind when

looking at the object? And why? Maybe there is a reason. Look for the reason but not too long. If you don't find the reason, forget it.

- Small supper.
- Nice talk (no complaints) 10 min. When nobody to talk with, phone or internet conversation oral or written.
- Walk 10 min.
- If you have the invading thoughts about eating, ask yourself if it is possible to ignore them.

Yes

Great! In such a case continue ignoring them.

No

You have to learn to ignore the invading thoughts.

This Guide will teach you to ignore the invading thoughts.

Remember: even if you cannot stop the invading thoughts, the invading thoughts cannot stop you to live a normal life.

If you believe in things which other people consider strange, try to keep your strange believes for yourself. Everybody has to make the selection of what can be told to other people and what must be private. Believe

me, many people have strange believes. Even much stranger than yours. And they are not considered to be sick. Why? Because they keep their strange believes for themselves. That is the secret.

***

Night

Before sleep

- Take a shower (warm water) 1 min.
- Small physical excercise 3 min.

In Bed

- Repeat STOP (10 times if you have invading thoughts).
- Say slowly whenever you are invaded by the thoughts about eating: sun, flower, seven, path, tee, run, yellow, apple, fish, rain, pen, water, smile, talk, life, sky.
- Think of three different words, any words which just come to your mind at the moment and make a simple story using these 3 words. Repeat untill you fall asleep.

If you cannot fall asleep

- Say slowly whenever you are invaded by the thoughts about eating: sun, flower, seven, path,

tee, run, yellow, apple, fish, rain, pen, water, smile, talk, life, sky.

If you cannot asleep

- Think of three different words, any words which just come to your mind at the moment and make a simple story using these 3 words. Repeat untill you fall asleep.

If above does not help

- Stand up and go to the toilet (when possible with as little light as possible)
- Say slowly whenever you are invaded by the thoughts about eating: sun, flower, seven, path, tee, run, yellow, apple, fish, rain, pen, water, smile, talk, life, sky.
- Think of three different words, any words which just come to your mind at the moment and make a simple story using these 3 words. Repeat untill you fall asleep.

If above does not help

- Say STOP untill you fall asleep

If above does not help

- Go to the kitchen and have a very small snack.

- Back to the bed think of three different words, any words which just come to your mind at the moment and make a simple story using these 3 words. Repeat untill you fall asleep.
- If above does not help think of three different words, any words which just come to your mind at the moment and make a simple story using these 3 words. Repeat untill you fall asleep.
- Say slowly whenever you are invaded by the thoughts about eating: sun, flower, seven, path, tee, run, yellow, apple, fish, rain, pen, water, smile, talk, life, sky. Repeat untill you fall asleep.

***

Week Two

***

Day 1

Morning

* Say STOP whenever thoughts about eating come to your mind.

* Say slowly whenever you are invaded by the thoughts about eating: sun, flower, seven, path, tee, run, yellow, apple, fish, rain, pen, water, smile, talk, life, sky.

* If above does not help to stop the thoughts about eating just turn your attention away from the invading thoughts about eating. The best way to turn your attention away from the invading thoughts about eating in your head is by doing one of your favorite occupations. Do not be ashamed of any occupation to turn your attention away from the invading thoughts in your head. ALWAYS be busy with your favorite occupation when unsupportable thoughts come to your head.

* Be careful to keep for yourself these of your believes which are found to be strange by the people.

* CONTROL what you say. Say only things which are not strange for the people. You surely already know which of your believes are found to be strange by the people.

* If you do not know yet which of your believes are found to be strange by the people, OBSERVE how people react on what you say. If you see that people are ALERTED by your believes, it means your believes are strange. From now on AVOID presenting such believes.

* Think of three different words, any words which just come to your mind at the moment and make a simple story using these 3 words. Repeat 3 times.

* Try to concentrate on an object close to you, any object. What do you feel when looking at the object? What thoughts come to your mind when looking at the object? And why? Maybe there is a reason. Look for the reason but not too long. If you don't find the reason, forget it.

* Small physical excercise (10 min)

* Small breakfast.

* Nice talk (no complaints, no problematic questions) 10 min. When nobody to talk with, phone or internet conversation oral or written.

* Walk 15 min.

* If you have invading thoughts about eating, ask yourself if it is possible to ignore them.

Yes

Great! In such a case continue ignoring them.

No

You have to learn to ignore the invading thoughts about eating.

This Guide will teach you to ignore the invading thoughts about eating.

Remember: even if you cannot stop the invading thoughts, the invading thoughts cannot stop you to live a normal life.

If you believe in things which other people consider strange, try to keep your strange believes for yourself. Everybody has to make the selection of what can be told to other people and what must be private. Believe me, many people have strange believes. Even much stranger than yours. And they are not considered to be sick. Why? Because they keep their strange believes for themselves. That is the secret.

***

Afternoon

* Say slowly whenever you are invaded by the thoughts about eating: sun, flower, seven, path, tee, run, yellow, apple, fish, rain, pen, water, smile, talk, life, sky.

* Think of three different words, any words which just come to your mind at the moment and make a simple story using these 3 words. Repeat 3 times.

* Try to concentrate on an object close to you, any object. What do you feel when looking at the object? What thoughts come to your mind when looking at the

object? And why? Maybe there is a reason. Look for the reason but not too long. If you don't find the reason, forget it.

* Dinner and half an hour break (you can sleep).

* Nice talk (no complaints) 15 min. When nobody to talk with, phone or internet conversation oral or written.

* Walk 20 min.

* If you have the invading thoughts about eating, ask yourself if it is possible to ignore them.

Yes

Great! In such a case continue ignoring them.

No

You have to learn to ignore the invading thoughts.

This Guide will teach you to ignore the invading thoughts about eating.

Remember: even if you cannot stop the invading thoughts, the invading thoughts cannot stop you to live a normal life.

If you believe in things which other people consider strange, try to keep your strange believes for yourself. Everybody has to make the selection of what can be

told to other people and what must be private. Believe me, many people have strange believes. Even much stranger than yours. And they are not considered to be sick. Why? Because they keep their strange believes for themselves. That is the secret.

***

Evening

- Say slowly whenever you are invaded by the thoughts about eating: sun, flower, seven, path, tee, run, yellow, apple, fish, rain, pen, water, smile, talk, life, sky.

- Think of three different words, any words which just come to your mind at the moment and make a simple story using these 3 words. Repeat 3 times.
  - Try to concentrate on an object close to you, any object. What do you feel when looking at the object? What thoughts come to your mind when looking at the object? And why? Maybe there is a reason. Look for the reason but not too long. If you don't find the reason, forget it.
  - Small supper.
  - Nice talk (no complaints) 10 min. When nobody to talk with, phone or internet conversation oral or written.

- Walk 10 min.
- If you have the invading thoughts about eating, ask yourself if it is possible to ignore them.

Yes

Great! In such a case continue ignoring them.

No

You have to learn to ignore the invading thoughts.

This Guide will teach you to ignore the invading thoughts.

Remember: even if you cannot stop the invading thoughts, the invading thoughts cannot stop you to live a normal life.

If you believe in things which other people consider strange, try to keep your strange believes for yourself. Everybody has to make the selection of what can be told to other people and what must be private. Believe me, many people have strange believes. Even much stranger than yours. And they are not considered to be sick. Why? Because they keep their strange believes for themselves. That is the secret.

***

Night

Before sleep

- Take a shower (warm water) 1 min.
- Small physical excercise 3 min.

In Bed

- Repeat STOP (10 times if you have invading thoughts).
- Say slowly whenever you are invaded by the thoughts about eating: sun, flower, seven, path, tee, run, yellow, apple, fish, rain, pen, water, smile, talk, life, sky.
- Think of three different words, any words which just come to your mind at the moment and make a simple story using these 3 words. Repeat untill you fall asleep.

If you cannot fall asleep

- Say slowly whenever you are invaded by the thoughts about eating: sun, flower, seven, path, tee, run, yellow, apple, fish, rain, pen, water, smile, talk, life, sky.

If you cannot asleep

- Think of three different words, any words which just come to your mind at the moment and make a simple story using these 3 words. Repeat untill you fall asleep.

If above does not help

- Stand up and go to the toilet (when possible with as little light as possible)
- Say slowly whenever you are invaded by the thoughts about eating: sun, flower, seven, path, tee, run, yellow, apple, fish, rain, pen, water, smile, talk, life, sky.
- Think of three different words, any words which just come to your mind at the moment and make a simple story using these 3 words. Repeat untill you fall asleep.

If above does not help

- Say STOP untill you fall asleep

If above does not help

- Go to the kitchen and have a very small snack.
- Back to the bed think of three different words, any words which just come to your mind at the moment and make a simple story using these 3 words. Repeat untill you fall asleep.
- If above does not help think of three different words, any words which just come to your mind at the moment and make a simple story using these 3 words. Repeat untill you fall asleep.

- Say slowly whenever you are invaded by the thoughts about eating: sun, flower, seven, path, tee, run, yellow, apple, fish, rain, pen, water, smile, talk, life, sky. Repeat untill you fall asleep.

***

Day 2

Morning

* Say STOP whenever thoughts about eating come to your mind.

* Say slowly whenever you are invaded by the thoughts about eating: sun, flower, seven, path, tee, run, yellow, apple, fish, rain, pen, water, smile, talk, life, sky.

* If above does not help to stop the thoughts about eating just turn your attention away from the invading thoughts about eating. The best way to turn your attention away from the invading thoughts about eating in your head is by doing one of your favorite occupations. Do not be ashamed of any occupation to turn your attention away from the invading thoughts in your head. ALWAYS be busy with your favorite occupation when unsupportable thoughts come to your head.

* Be careful to keep for yourself these of your believes which are found to be strange by the people.

* CONTROL what you say. Say only things which are not strange for the people. You surely already know which of your believes are found to be strange by the people.

* If you do not know yet which of your believes are found to be strange by the people, OBSERVE how people react on what you say. If you see that people are ALERTED by your believes, it means your believes are strange. From now on AVOID presenting such believes.

* Think of three different words, any words which just come to your mind at the moment and make a simple story using these 3 words. Repeat 3 times.

* Try to concentrate on an object close to you, any object. What do you feel when looking at the object? What thoughts come to your mind when looking at the object? And why?Maybe there is a reason. Look for the reason but not too long. If you don't find the reason, forget it.

* Small physical excercise (10 min)

* Small breakfast.

* Nice talk (no complaints, no problematic questions) 10 min. When nobody to talk with, phone or internet conversation oral or written.

* Walk 15 min.

* If you have invading thoughts about eating, ask yourself if it is possible to ignore them.

Yes

Great! In such a case continue ignoring them.

No

You have to learn to ignore the invading thoughts about eating.

This Guide will teach you to ignore the invading thoughts about eating.

Remember: even if you cannot stop the invading thoughts, the invading thoughts cannot stop you to live a normal life.

If you believe in things which other people consider strange, try to keep your strange believes for yourself. Everybody has to make the selection of what can be told to other people and what must be private. Believe me, many people have strange believes. Even much stranger than yours. And they are not considered to be

sick. Why? Because they keep their strange believes for themselves. That is the secret.

***

Afternoon

* Say slowly whenever you are invaded by the thoughts about eating: sun, flower, seven, path, tee, run, yellow, apple, fish, rain, pen, water, smile, talk, life, sky.

* Think of three different words, any words which just come to your mind at the moment and make a simple story using these 3 words. Repeat 3 times.

* Try to concentrate on an object close to you, any object. What do you feel when looking at the object? What thoughts come to your mind when looking at the object? And why?Maybe there is a reason. Look for the reason but not too long. If you don't find the reason, forget it.

* Dinner and half an hour break (you can sleep).

* Nice talk (no complaints) 15 min. When nobody to talk with, phone or internet conversation oral or written.

* Walk 20 min.

* If you have the invading thoughts about eating, ask yourself if it is possible to ignore them.

Yes

Great! In such a case continue ignoring them.

No

You have to learn to ignore the invading thoughts.

This Guide will teach you to ignore the invading thoughts about eating.

Remember: even if you cannot stop the invading thoughts, the invading thoughts cannot stop you to live a normal life.

If you believe in things which other people consider strange, try to keep your strange believes for yourself. Everybody has to make the selection of what can be told to other people and what must be private. Believe me, many people have strange believes. Even much stranger than yours. And they are not considered to be sick. Why? Because they keep their strange believes for themselves. That is the secret.

***

Evening

- Say slowly whenever you are invaded by the thoughts about eating: sun, flower, seven, path, tee, run, yellow, apple, fish, rain, pen, water, smile, talk, life, sky.

- Think of three different words, any words which just come to your mind at the moment and make a simple story using these 3 words. Repeat 3 times.
  - Try to concentrate on an object close to you, any object. What do you feel when looking at the object? What thoughts come to your mind when looking at the object? And why? Maybe there is a reason. Look for the reason but not too long. If you don't find the reason, forget it.
  - Small supper.
  - Nice talk (no complaints) 10 min. When nobody to talk with, phone or internet conversation oral or written.
  - Walk 10 min.
  - If you have the invading thoughts about eating, ask yourself if it is possible to ignore them.

Yes

Great! In such a case continue ignoring them.

No

You have to learn to ignore the invading thoughts.

This Guide will teach you to ignore the invading thoughts.

Remember: even if you cannot stop the invading thoughts, the invading thoughts cannot stop you to live a normal life.

If you believe in things which other people consider strange, try to keep your strange believes for yourself. Everybody has to make the selection of what can be told to other people and what must be private. Believe me, many people have strange believes. Even much stranger than yours. And they are not considered to be sick. Why? Because they keep their strange believes for themselves. That is the secret.

***

Night

Before sleep

- Take a shower (warm water) 1 min.
- Small physical excercise 3 min.

In Bed

- Repeat STOP (10 times if you have invading thoughts).

- Say slowly whenever you are invaded by the thoughts about eating: sun, flower, seven, path, tee, run, yellow, apple, fish, rain, pen, water, smile, talk, life, sky.
- Think of three different words, any words which just come to your mind at the moment and make a simple story using these 3 words. Repeat untill you fall asleep.

If you cannot fall asleep

- Say slowly whenever you are invaded by the thoughts about eating: sun, flower, seven, path, tee, run, yellow, apple, fish, rain, pen, water, smile, talk, life, sky.

If you cannot asleep

- Think of three different words, any words which just come to your mind at the moment and make a simple story using these 3 words. Repeat untill you fall asleep.

If above does not help

- Stand up and go to the toilet (when possible with as little light as possible)
- Say slowly whenever you are invaded by the thoughts about eating: sun, flower, seven, path,

tee, run, yellow, apple, fish, rain, pen, water, smile, talk, life, sky.
- Think of three different words, any words which just come to your mind at the moment and make a simple story using these 3 words. Repeat untill you fall asleep.

If above does not help
- Say STOP untill you fall asleep

If above does not help
- Go to the kitchen and have a very small snack.
- Back to the bed think of three different words, any words which just come to your mind at the moment and make a simple story using these 3 words. Repeat untill you fall asleep.
- If above does not help think of three different words, any words which just come to your mind at the moment and make a simple story using these 3 words. Repeat untill you fall asleep.
- Say slowly whenever you are invaded by the thoughts about eating: sun, flower, seven, path, tee, run, yellow, apple, fish, rain, pen, water, smile, talk, life, sky. Repeat untill you fall asleep.

***

Day 3

Morning

* Say STOP whenever thoughts about eating come to your mind.

* Say slowly whenever you are invaded by the thoughts about eating: sun, flower, seven, path, tee, run, yellow, apple, fish, rain, pen, water, smile, talk, life, sky.

* If above does not help to stop the thoughts about eating just turn your attention away from the invading thoughts about eating. The best way to turn your attention away from the invading thoughts about eating in your head is by doing one of your favorite occupations. Do not be ashamed of any occupation to turn your attention away from the invading thoughts in your head. ALWAYS be busy with your favorite occupation when unsupportable thoughts come to your head.

* Be careful to keep for yourself these of your believes which are found to be strange by the people.

* CONTROL what you say. Say only things which are not strange for the people. You surely already know which of your believes are found to be strange by the people.

* If you do not know yet which of your believes are found to be strange by the people, OBSERVE how

people react on what you say. If you see that people are ALERTED by your believes, it means your believes are strange. From now on AVOID presenting such believes.

* Think of three different words, any words which just come to your mind at the moment and make a simple story using these 3 words. Repeat 3 times.

* Try to concentrate on an object close to you, any object. What do you feel when looking at the object? What thoughts come to your mind when looking at the object? And why? Maybe there is a reason. Look for the reason but not too long. If you don't find the reason, forget it.

* Small physical excercise (10 min)

* Small breakfast.

* Nice talk (no complaints, no problematic questions) 10 min. When nobody to talk with, phone or internet conversation oral or written.

* Walk 15 min.

* If you have invading thoughts about eating, ask yourself if it is possible to ignore them.

Yes

Great! In such a case continue ignoring them.

No

You have to learn to ignore the invading thoughts about eating.

This Guide will teach you to ignore the invading thoughts about eating.

Remember: even if you cannot stop the invading thoughts, the invading thoughts cannot stop you to live a normal life.

If you believe in things which other people consider strange, try to keep your strange believes for yourself. Everybody has to make the selection of what can be told to other people and what must be private. Believe me, many people have strange believes. Even much stranger than yours. And they are not considered to be sick. Why? Because they keep their strange believes for themselves. That is the secret.

***

Afternoon

* Say slowly whenever you are invaded by the thoughts about eating: sun, flower, seven, path, tee, run, yellow, apple, fish, rain, pen, water, smile, talk, life, sky.

* Think of three different words, any words which just come to your mind at the moment and make a simple story using these 3 words. Repeat 3 times.

* Try to concentrate on an object close to you, any object. What do you feel when looking at the object? What thoughts come to your mind when looking at the object? And why? Maybe there is a reason. Look for the reason but not too long. If you don't find the reason, forget it.

* Dinner and half an hour break (you can sleep).

* Nice talk (no complaints) 15 min. When nobody to talk with, phone or internet conversation oral or written.

* Walk 20 min.

* If you have the invading thoughts about eating, ask yourself if it is possible to ignore them.

Yes

Great! In such a case continue ignoring them.

No

You have to learn to ignore the invading thoughts.

This Guide will teach you to ignore the invading thoughts about eating.

Remember: even if you cannot stop the invading thoughts, the invading thoughts cannot stop you to live a normal life.

If you believe in things which other people consider strange, try to keep your strange believes for yourself. Everybody has to make the selection of what can be told to other people and what must be private. Believe me, many people have strange believes. Even much stranger than yours. And they are not considered to be sick. Why? Because they keep their strange believes for themselves. That is the secret.

***

Evening

- Say slowly whenever you are invaded by the thoughts about eating: sun, flower, seven, path, tee, run, yellow, apple, fish, rain, pen, water, smile, talk, life, sky.

- Think of three different words, any words which just come to your mind at the moment and make a simple story using these 3 words. Repeat 3 times.
  - Try to concentrate on an object close to you, any object. What do you feel when looking at the object? What thoughts come to your mind when

looking at the object? And why? Maybe there is a reason. Look for the reason but not too long. If you don't find the reason, forget it.

- Small supper.
- Nice talk (no complaints) 10 min. When nobody to talk with, phone or internet conversation oral or written.
- Walk 10 min.
- If you have the invading thoughts about eating, ask yourself if it is possible to ignore them.

Yes

Great! In such a case continue ignoring them.

No

You have to learn to ignore the invading thoughts.

This Guide will teach you to ignore the invading thoughts.

Remember: even if you cannot stop the invading thoughts, the invading thoughts cannot stop you to live a normal life.

If you believe in things which other people consider strange, try to keep your strange believes for yourself. Everybody has to make the selection of what can be told to other people and what must be private. Believe

me, many people have strange believes. Even much stranger than yours. And they are not considered to be sick. Why? Because they keep their strange believes for themselves. That is the secret.

***

Night

Before sleep

- Take a shower (warm water) 1 min.
- Small physical excercise 3 min.

In Bed

- Repeat STOP (10 times if you have invading thoughts).
- Say slowly whenever you are invaded by the thoughts about eating: sun, flower, seven, path, tee, run, yellow, apple, fish, rain, pen, water, smile, talk, life, sky.
- Think of three different words, any words which just come to your mind at the moment and make a simple story using these 3 words. Repeat untill you fall asleep.

If you cannot fall asleep

- Say slowly whenever you are invaded by the thoughts about eating: sun, flower, seven, path,

tee, run, yellow, apple, fish, rain, pen, water, smile, talk, life, sky.

If you cannot asleep

- Think of three different words, any words which just come to your mind at the moment and make a simple story using these 3 words. Repeat untill you fall asleep.

If above does not help

- Stand up and go to the toilet (when possible with as little light as possible)
- Say slowly whenever you are invaded by the thoughts about eating: sun, flower, seven, path, tee, run, yellow, apple, fish, rain, pen, water, smile, talk, life, sky.
- Think of three different words, any words which just come to your mind at the moment and make a simple story using these 3 words. Repeat untill you fall asleep.

If above does not help

- Say STOP untill you fall asleep

If above does not help

- Go to the kitchen and have a very small snack.

- Back to the bed think of three different words, any words which just come to your mind at the moment and make a simple story using these 3 words. Repeat untill you fall asleep.
- If above does not help think of three different words, any words which just come to your mind at the moment and make a simple story using these 3 words. Repeat untill you fall asleep.
- Say slowly whenever you are invaded by the thoughts about eating: sun, flower, seven, path, tee, run, yellow, apple, fish, rain, pen, water, smile, talk, life, sky. Repeat untill you fall asleep.

***

Day 4

Morning

* Say STOP whenever thoughts about eating come to your mind.

* Say slowly whenever you are invaded by the thoughts about eating: sun, flower, seven, path, tee, run, yellow, apple, fish, rain, pen, water, smile, talk, life, sky.

* If above does not help to stop the thoughts about eating just turn your attention away from the invading thoughts about eating. The best way to turn your

attention away from the invading thoughts about eating in your head is by doing one of your favorite occupations. Do not be ashamed of any occupation to turn your attention away from the invading thoughts in your head. ALWAYS be busy with your favorite occupation when unsupportable thoughts come to your head.

* Be careful to keep for yourself these of your believes which are found to be strange by the people.

* CONTROL what you say. Say only things which are not strange for the people. You surely already know which of your believes are found to be strange by the people.

* If you do not know yet which of your believes are found to be strange by the people, OBSERVE how people react on what you say. If you see that people are ALERTED by your believes, it means your believes are strange. From now on AVOID presenting such believes.

* Think of three different words, any words which just come to your mind at the moment and make a simple story using these 3 words. Repeat 3 times.

* Try to concentrate on an object close to you, any object. What do you feel when looking at the object? What thoughts come to your mind when looking at the object? And why?Maybe there is a reason. Look for the

reason but not too long. If you don't find the reason, forget it.

* Small physical excercise (10 min)

* Small breakfast.

* Nice talk (no complaints, no problematic questions) 10 min. When nobody to talk with, phone or internet conversation oral or written.

* Walk 15 min.

* If you have invading thoughts about eating, ask yourself if it is possible to ignore them.

Yes

Great! In such a case continue ignoring them.

No

You have to learn to ignore the invading thoughts about eating.

This Guide will teach you to ignore the invading thoughts about eating.

Remember: even if you cannot stop the invading thoughts, the invading thoughts cannot stop you to live a normal life.

If you believe in things which other people consider strange, try to keep your strange believes for yourself. Everybody has to make the selection of what can be told to other people and what must be private. Believe me, many people have strange believes. Even much stranger than yours. And they are not considered to be sick. Why? Because they keep their strange believes for themselves. That is the secret.

***

Afternoon

* Say slowly whenever you are invaded by the thoughts about eating: sun, flower, seven, path, tee, run, yellow, apple, fish, rain, pen, water, smile, talk, life, sky.

* Think of three different words, any words which just come to your mind at the moment and make a simple story using these 3 words. Repeat 3 times.

* Try to concentrate on an object close to you, any object. What do you feel when looking at the object? What thoughts come to your mind when looking at the object? And why? Maybe there is a reason. Look for the reason but not too long. If you don't find the reason, forget it.

* Dinner and half an hour break (you can sleep).

* Nice talk (no complaints) 15 min. When nobody to talk with, phone or internet conversation oral or written.

* Walk 20 min.

* If you have the invading thoughts about eating, ask yourself if it is possible to ignore them.

Yes

Great! In such a case continue ignoring them.

No

You have to learn to ignore the invading thoughts.

This Guide will teach you to ignore the invading thoughts about eating.

Remember: even if you cannot stop the invading thoughts, the invading thoughts cannot stop you to live a normal life.

If you believe in things which other people consider strange, try to keep your strange believes for yourself. Everybody has to make the selection of what can be told to other people and what must be private. Believe me, many people have strange believes. Even much stranger than yours. And they are not considered to be

sick. Why? Because they keep their strange believes for themselves. That is the secret.

***

Evening

- Say slowly whenever you are invaded by the thoughts about eating: sun, flower, seven, path, tee, run, yellow, apple, fish, rain, pen, water, smile, talk, life, sky.

- Think of three different words, any words which just come to your mind at the moment and make a simple story using these 3 words. Repeat 3 times.
  - Try to concentrate on an object close to you, any object. What do you feel when looking at the object? What thoughts come to your mind when looking at the object? And why? Maybe there is a reason. Look for the reason but not too long. If you don't find the reason, forget it.
  - Small supper.
  - Nice talk (no complaints) 10 min. When nobody to talk with, phone or internet conversation oral or written.
  - Walk 10 min.
  - If you have the invading thoughts about eating, ask yourself if it is possible to ignore them.

Yes

Great! In such a case continue ignoring them.

No

You have to learn to ignore the invading thoughts.

This Guide will teach you to ignore the invading thoughts.

Remember: even if you cannot stop the invading thoughts, the invading thoughts cannot stop you to live a normal life.

If you believe in things which other people consider strange, try to keep your strange believes for yourself. Everybody has to make the selection of what can be told to other people and what must be private. Believe me, many people have strange believes. Even much stranger than yours. And they are not considered to be sick. Why? Because they keep their strange believes for themselves. That is the secret.

***

Night

Before sleep

- Take a shower (warm water) 1 min.
- Small physical excercise 3 min.

In Bed

- Repeat STOP (10 times if you have invading thoughts).
- Say slowly whenever you are invaded by the thoughts about eating: sun, flower, seven, path, tee, run, yellow, apple, fish, rain, pen, water, smile, talk, life, sky.
- Think of three different words, any words which just come to your mind at the moment and make a simple story using these 3 words. Repeat untill you fall asleep.

If you cannot fall asleep

- Say slowly whenever you are invaded by the thoughts about eating: sun, flower, seven, path, tee, run, yellow, apple, fish, rain, pen, water, smile, talk, life, sky.

If you cannot asleep

- Think of three different words, any words which just come to your mind at the moment and make a simple story using these 3 words. Repeat untill you fall asleep.

If above does not help

- Stand up and go to the toilet (when possible with as little light as possible)

- Say slowly whenever you are invaded by the thoughts about eating: sun, flower, seven, path, tee, run, yellow, apple, fish, rain, pen, water, smile, talk, life, sky.
- Think of three different words, any words which just come to your mind at the moment and make a simple story using these 3 words. Repeat untill you fall asleep.

If above does not help

- Say STOP untill you fall asleep

If above does not help

- Go to the kitchen and have a very small snack.
- Back to the bed think of three different words, any words which just come to your mind at the moment and make a simple story using these 3 words. Repeat untill you fall asleep.
- If above does not help think of three different words, any words which just come to your mind at the moment and make a simple story using these 3 words. Repeat untill you fall asleep.
- Say slowly whenever you are invaded by the thoughts about eating: sun, flower, seven, path, tee, run, yellow, apple, fish, rain, pen, water, smile, talk, life, sky. Repeat untill you fall asleep.

***

Day 5

Morning

* Say STOP whenever thoughts about eating come to your mind.

* Say slowly whenever you are invaded by the thoughts about eating: sun, flower, seven, path, tee, run, yellow, apple, fish, rain, pen, water, smile, talk, life, sky.

* If above does not help to stop the thoughts about eating just turn your attention away from the invading thoughts about eating. The best way to turn your attention away from the invading thoughts about eating in your head is by doing one of your favorite occupations. Do not be ashamed of any occupation to turn your attention away from the invading thoughts in your head. ALWAYS be busy with your favorite occupation when unsupportable thoughts come to your head.

* Be careful to keep for yourself these of your believes which are found to be strange by the people.

* CONTROL what you say. Say only things which are not strange for the people. You surely already know which of your believes are found to be strange by the people.

* If you do not know yet which of your believes are found to be strange by the people, OBSERVE how people react on what you say. If you see that people are ALERTED by your believes, it means your believes are strange. From now on AVOID presenting such believes.

* Think of three different words, any words which just come to your mind at the moment and make a simple story using these 3 words. Repeat 3 times.

* Try to concentrate on an object close to you, any object. What do you feel when looking at the object? What thoughts come to your mind when looking at the object? And why? Maybe there is a reason. Look for the reason but not too long. If you don't find the reason, forget it.

* Small physical excercise (10 min)

* Small breakfast.

* Nice talk (no complaints, no problematic questions) 10 min. When nobody to talk with, phone or internet conversation oral or written.

* Walk 15 min.

* If you have invading thoughts about eating, ask yourself if it is possible to ignore them.

Yes

Great! In such a case continue ignoring them.

No

You have to learn to ignore the invading thoughts about eating.

This Guide will teach you to ignore the invading thoughts about eating.

Remember: even if you cannot stop the invading thoughts, the invading thoughts cannot stop you to live a normal life.

If you believe in things which other people consider strange, try to keep your strange believes for yourself. Everybody has to make the selection of what can be told to other people and what must be private. Believe me, many people have strange believes. Even much stranger than yours. And they are not considered to be sick. Why? Because they keep their strange believes for themselves. That is the secret.

***

Afternoon

* Say slowly whenever you are invaded by the thoughts about eating: sun, flower, seven, path, tee, run, yellow, apple, fish, rain, pen, water, smile, talk, life, sky.

* Think of three different words, any words which just come to your mind at the moment and make a simple story using these 3 words. Repeat 3 times.

* Try to concentrate on an object close to you, any object. What do you feel when looking at the object? What thoughts come to your mind when looking at the object? And why? Maybe there is a reason. Look for the reason but not too long. If you don't find the reason, forget it.

* Dinner and half an hour break (you can sleep).

* Nice talk (no complaints) 15 min. When nobody to talk with, phone or internet conversation oral or written.

* Walk 20 min.

* If you have the invading thoughts about eating, ask yourself if it is possible to ignore them.

Yes

Great! In such a case continue ignoring them.

No

You have to learn to ignore the invading thoughts.

This Guide will teach you to ignore the invading thoughts about eating.

Remember: even if you cannot stop the invading thoughts, the invading thoughts cannot stop you to live a normal life.

If you believe in things which other people consider strange, try to keep your strange believes for yourself. Everybody has to make the selection of what can be told to other people and what must be private. Believe me, many people have strange believes. Even much stranger than yours. And they are not considered to be sick. Why? Because they keep their strange believes for themselves. That is the secret.

***

Evening

- Say slowly whenever you are invaded by the thoughts about eating: sun, flower, seven, path, tee, run, yellow, apple, fish, rain, pen, water, smile, talk, life, sky.

- Think of three different words, any words which just come to your mind at the moment and make a simple story using these 3 words. Repeat 3 times.

- Try to concentrate on an object close to you, any object. What do you feel when looking at the object? What thoughts come to your mind when looking at the object? And why? Maybe there is a reason. Look for the reason but not too long. If you don't find the reason, forget it.
- Small supper.
- Nice talk (no complaints) 10 min. When nobody to talk with, phone or internet conversation oral or written.
- Walk 10 min.
- If you have the invading thoughts about eating, ask yourself if it is possible to ignore them.

Yes

Great! In such a case continue ignoring them.

No

You have to learn to ignore the invading thoughts.

This Guide will teach you to ignore the invading thoughts.

Remember: even if you cannot stop the invading thoughts, the invading thoughts cannot stop you to live a normal life.

If you believe in things which other people consider strange, try to keep your strange believes for yourself. Everybody has to make the selection of what can be told to other people and what must be private. Believe me, many people have strange believes. Even much stranger than yours. And they are not considered to be sick. Why? Because they keep their strange believes for themselves. That is the secret.

***

Night

Before sleep

- Take a shower (warm water) 1 min.
- Small physical excercise 3 min.

In Bed

- Repeat STOP (10 times if you have invading thoughts).
- Say slowly whenever you are invaded by the thoughts about eating: sun, flower, seven, path, tee, run, yellow, apple, fish, rain, pen, water, smile, talk, life, sky.
- Think of three different words, any words which just come to your mind at the moment and make a simple story using these 3 words. Repeat untill you fall asleep.

If you cannot fall asleep

- Say slowly whenever you are invaded by the thoughts about eating: sun, flower, seven, path, tee, run, yellow, apple, fish, rain, pen, water, smile, talk, life, sky.

If you cannot asleep

- Think of three different words, any words which just come to your mind at the moment and make a simple story using these 3 words. Repeat untill you fall asleep.

If above does not help

- Stand up and go to the toilet (when possible with as little light as possible)
- Say slowly whenever you are invaded by the thoughts about eating: sun, flower, seven, path, tee, run, yellow, apple, fish, rain, pen, water, smile, talk, life, sky.
- Think of three different words, any words which just come to your mind at the moment and make a simple story using these 3 words. Repeat untill you fall asleep.

If above does not help

- Say STOP untill you fall asleep

If above does not help

- Go to the kitchen and have a very small snack.
- Back to the bed think of three different words, any words which just come to your mind at the moment and make a simple story using these 3 words. Repeat untill you fall asleep.
- If above does not help think of three different words, any words which just come to your mind at the moment and make a simple story using these 3 words. Repeat untill you fall asleep.
- Say slowly whenever you are invaded by the thoughts about eating: sun, flower, seven, path, tee, run, yellow, apple, fish, rain, pen, water, smile, talk, life, sky. Repeat untill you fall asleep.

***

Day 6

Morning

* Say STOP whenever thoughts about eating come to your mind.

* Say slowly whenever you are invaded by the thoughts about eating: sun, flower, seven, path, tee, run, yellow, apple, fish, rain, pen, water, smile, talk, life, sky.

* If above does not help to stop the thoughts about eating just turn your attention away from the invading thoughts about eating. The best way to turn your attention away from the invading thoughts about eating in your head is by doing one of your favorite occupations. Do not be ashamed of any occupation to turn your attention away from the invading thoughts in your head. ALWAYS be busy with your favorite occupation when unsupportable thoughts come to your head.

* Be careful to keep for yourself these of your believes which are found to be strange by the people.

* CONTROL what you say. Say only things which are not strange for the people. You surely already know which of your believes are found to be strange by the people.

* If you do not know yet which of your believes are found to be strange by the people, OBSERVE how people react on what you say. If you see that people are ALERTED by your believes, it means your believes are strange. From now on AVOID presenting such believes.

* Think of three different words, any words which just come to your mind at the moment and make a simple story using these 3 words. Repeat 3 times.

* Try to concentrate on an object close to you, any object. What do you feel when looking at the object? What thoughts come to your mind when looking at the object? And why? Maybe there is a reason. Look for the reason but not too long. If you don't find the reason, forget it.

* Small physical excercise (10 min)

* Small breakfast.

* Nice talk (no complaints, no problematic questions) 10 min. When nobody to talk with, phone or internet conversation oral or written.

* Walk 15 min.

* If you have invading thoughts about eating, ask yourself if it is possible to ignore them.

Yes

Great! In such a case continue ignoring them.

No

You have to learn to ignore the invading thoughts about eating.

This Guide will teach you to ignore the invading thoughts about eating.

Remember: even if you cannot stop the invading thoughts, the invading thoughts cannot stop you to live a normal life.

If you believe in things which other people consider strange, try to keep your strange believes for yourself. Everybody has to make the selection of what can be told to other people and what must be private. Believe me, many people have strange believes. Even much stranger than yours. And they are not considered to be sick. Why? Because they keep their strange believes for themselves. That is the secret.

***

Afternoon

* Say slowly whenever you are invaded by the thoughts about eating: sun, flower, seven, path, tee, run, yellow, apple, fish, rain, pen, water, smile, talk, life, sky.

* Think of three different words, any words which just come to your mind at the moment and make a simple story using these 3 words. Repeat 3 times.

* Try to concentrate on an object close to you, any object. What do you feel when looking at the object? What thoughts come to your mind when looking at the

object? And why? Maybe there is a reason. Look for the reason but not too long. If you don't find the reason, forget it.

* Dinner and half an hour break (you can sleep).

* Nice talk (no complaints) 15 min. When nobody to talk with, phone or internet conversation oral or written.

* Walk 20 min.

* If you have the invading thoughts about eating, ask yourself if it is possible to ignore them.

Yes

Great! In such a case continue ignoring them.

No

You have to learn to ignore the invading thoughts.

This Guide will teach you to ignore the invading thoughts about eating.

Remember: even if you cannot stop the invading thoughts, the invading thoughts cannot stop you to live a normal life.

If you believe in things which other people consider strange, try to keep your strange believes for yourself. Everybody has to make the selection of what can be

told to other people and what must be private. Believe me, many people have strange believes. Even much stranger than yours. And they are not considered to be sick. Why? Because they keep their strange believes for themselves. That is the secret.

***

Evening

- Say slowly whenever you are invaded by the thoughts about eating: sun, flower, seven, path, tee, run, yellow, apple, fish, rain, pen, water, smile, talk, life, sky.

- Think of three different words, any words which just come to your mind at the moment and make a simple story using these 3 words. Repeat 3 times.
  - Try to concentrate on an object close to you, any object. What do you feel when looking at the object? What thoughts come to your mind when looking at the object? And why? Maybe there is a reason. Look for the reason but not too long. If you don't find the reason, forget it.
  - Small supper.
  - Nice talk (no complaints) 10 min. When nobody to talk with, phone or internet conversation oral or written.

- Walk 10 min.
- If you have the invading thoughts about eating, ask yourself if it is possible to ignore them.

Yes

Great! In such a case continue ignoring them.

No

You have to learn to ignore the invading thoughts.

This Guide will teach you to ignore the invading thoughts.

Remember: even if you cannot stop the invading thoughts, the invading thoughts cannot stop you to live a normal life.

If you believe in things which other people consider strange, try to keep your strange believes for yourself. Everybody has to make the selection of what can be told to other people and what must be private. Believe me, many people have strange believes. Even much stranger than yours. And they are not considered to be sick. Why? Because they keep their strange believes for themselves. That is the secret.

***

Night

Before sleep

- Take a shower (warm water) 1 min.
- Small physical excercise 3 min.

In Bed

- Repeat STOP (10 times if you have invading thoughts).
- Say slowly whenever you are invaded by the thoughts about eating: sun, flower, seven, path, tee, run, yellow, apple, fish, rain, pen, water, smile, talk, life, sky.
- Think of three different words, any words which just come to your mind at the moment and make a simple story using these 3 words. Repeat untill you fall asleep.

If you cannot fall asleep

- Say slowly whenever you are invaded by the thoughts about eating: sun, flower, seven, path, tee, run, yellow, apple, fish, rain, pen, water, smile, talk, life, sky.

If you cannot asleep

- Think of three different words, any words which just come to your mind at the moment and make a simple story using these 3 words. Repeat untill you fall asleep.

If above does not help

- Stand up and go to the toilet (when possible with as little light as possible)
- Say slowly whenever you are invaded by the thoughts about eating: sun, flower, seven, path, tee, run, yellow, apple, fish, rain, pen, water, smile, talk, life, sky.
- Think of three different words, any words which just come to your mind at the moment and make a simple story using these 3 words. Repeat untill you fall asleep.

If above does not help

- Say STOP untill you fall asleep

If above does not help

- Go to the kitchen and have a very small snack.
- Back to the bed think of three different words, any words which just come to your mind at the moment and make a simple story using these 3 words. Repeat untill you fall asleep.
- If above does not help think of three different words, any words which just come to your mind at the moment and make a simple story using these 3 words. Repeat untill you fall asleep.

- Say slowly whenever you are invaded by the thoughts about eating: sun, flower, seven, path, tee, run, yellow, apple, fish, rain, pen, water, smile, talk, life, sky. Repeat untill you fall asleep.

***

Day 7

Morning

* Say STOP whenever thoughts about eating come to your mind.

* Say slowly whenever you are invaded by the thoughts about eating: sun, flower, seven, path, tee, run, yellow, apple, fish, rain, pen, water, smile, talk, life, sky.

* If above does not help to stop the thoughts about eating just turn your attention away from the invading thoughts about eating. The best way to turn your attention away from the invading thoughts about eating in your head is by doing one of your favorite occupations. Do not be ashamed of any occupation to turn your attention away from the invading thoughts in your head. ALWAYS be busy with your favorite occupation when unsupportable thoughts come to your head.

* Be careful to keep for yourself these of your believes which are found to be strange by the people.

* CONTROL what you say. Say only things which are not strange for the people. You surely already know which of your believes are found to be strange by the people.

* If you do not know yet which of your believes are found to be strange by the people, OBSERVE how people react on what you say. If you see that people are ALERTED by your believes, it means your believes are strange. From now on AVOID presenting such believes.

* Think of three different words, any words which just come to your mind at the moment and make a simple story using these 3 words. Repeat 3 times.

* Try to concentrate on an object close to you, any object. What do you feel when looking at the object? What thoughts come to your mind when looking at the object? And why?Maybe there is a reason. Look for the reason but not too long. If you don't find the reason, forget it.

* Small physical excercise (10 min)

* Small breakfast.

* Nice talk (no complaints, no problematic questions) 10 min. When nobody to talk with, phone or internet conversation oral or written.

* Walk 15 min.

* If you have invading thoughts about eating, ask yourself if it is possible to ignore them.

Yes

Great! In such a case continue ignoring them.

No

You have to learn to ignore the invading thoughts about eating.

This Guide will teach you to ignore the invading thoughts about eating.

Remember: even if you cannot stop the invading thoughts, the invading thoughts cannot stop you to live a normal life.

If you believe in things which other people consider strange, try to keep your strange believes for yourself. Everybody has to make the selection of what can be told to other people and what must be private. Believe me, many people have strange believes. Even much stranger than yours. And they are not considered to be

sick. Why? Because they keep their strange believes for themselves. That is the secret.

***

Afternoon

* Say slowly whenever you are invaded by the thoughts about eating: sun, flower, seven, path, tee, run, yellow, apple, fish, rain, pen, water, smile, talk, life, sky.

* Think of three different words, any words which just come to your mind at the moment and make a simple story using these 3 words. Repeat 3 times.

* Try to concentrate on an object close to you, any object. What do you feel when looking at the object? What thoughts come to your mind when looking at the object? And why?Maybe there is a reason. Look for the reason but not too long. If you don't find the reason, forget it.

* Dinner and half an hour break (you can sleep).

* Nice talk (no complaints) 15 min. When nobody to talk with, phone or internet conversation oral or written.

* Walk 20 min.

* If you have the invading thoughts about eating, ask yourself if it is possible to ignore them.

Yes

Great! In such a case continue ignoring them.

No

You have to learn to ignore the invading thoughts.

This Guide will teach you to ignore the invading thoughts about eating.

Remember: even if you cannot stop the invading thoughts, the invading thoughts cannot stop you to live a normal life.

If you believe in things which other people consider strange, try to keep your strange believes for yourself. Everybody has to make the selection of what can be told to other people and what must be private. Believe me, many people have strange believes. Even much stranger than yours. And they are not considered to be sick. Why? Because they keep their strange believes for themselves. That is the secret.

***

Evening

- Say slowly whenever you are invaded by the thoughts about eating: sun, flower, seven, path, tee, run, yellow, apple, fish, rain, pen, water, smile, talk, life, sky.

- Think of three different words, any words which just come to your mind at the moment and make a simple story using these 3 words. Repeat 3 times.
  - Try to concentrate on an object close to you, any object. What do you feel when looking at the object? What thoughts come to your mind when looking at the object? And why? Maybe there is a reason. Look for the reason but not too long. If you don't find the reason, forget it.
  - Small supper.
  - Nice talk (no complaints) 10 min. When nobody to talk with, phone or internet conversation oral or written.
  - Walk 10 min.
  - If you have the invading thoughts about eating, ask yourself if it is possible to ignore them.

Yes

Great! In such a case continue ignoring them.

No

You have to learn to ignore the invading thoughts.

This Guide will teach you to ignore the invading thoughts.

Remember: even if you cannot stop the invading thoughts, the invading thoughts cannot stop you to live a normal life.

If you believe in things which other people consider strange, try to keep your strange believes for yourself. Everybody has to make the selection of what can be told to other people and what must be private. Believe me, many people have strange believes. Even much stranger than yours. And they are not considered to be sick. Why? Because they keep their strange believes for themselves. That is the secret.

***

Night

Before sleep

- Take a shower (warm water) 1 min.
- Small physical excercise 3 min.

In Bed

- Repeat STOP (10 times if you have invading thoughts).

- Say slowly whenever you are invaded by the thoughts about eating: sun, flower, seven, path, tee, run, yellow, apple, fish, rain, pen, water, smile, talk, life, sky.
- Think of three different words, any words which just come to your mind at the moment and make a simple story using these 3 words. Repeat untill you fall asleep.

If you cannot fall asleep

- Say slowly whenever you are invaded by the thoughts about eating: sun, flower, seven, path, tee, run, yellow, apple, fish, rain, pen, water, smile, talk, life, sky.

If you cannot asleep

- Think of three different words, any words which just come to your mind at the moment and make a simple story using these 3 words. Repeat untill you fall asleep.

If above does not help

- Stand up and go to the toilet (when possible with as little light as possible)
- Say slowly whenever you are invaded by the thoughts about eating: sun, flower, seven, path,

- tee, run, yellow, apple, fish, rain, pen, water, smile, talk, life, sky.
- Think of three different words, any words which just come to your mind at the moment and make a simple story using these 3 words. Repeat untill you fall asleep.

If above does not help

- Say STOP untill you fall asleep

If above does not help

- Go to the kitchen and have a very small snack.
- Back to the bed think of three different words, any words which just come to your mind at the moment and make a simple story using these 3 words. Repeat untill you fall asleep.
- If above does not help think of three different words, any words which just come to your mind at the moment and make a simple story using these 3 words. Repeat untill you fall asleep.
- Say slowly whenever you are invaded by the thoughts about eating: sun, flower, seven, path, tee, run, yellow, apple, fish, rain, pen, water, smile, talk, life, sky. Repeat untill you fall asleep.

***

Week Three

***

Day 1

Morning

* Say STOP whenever thoughts about eating come to your mind.

* Say slowly whenever you are invaded by the thoughts about eating: sun, flower, seven, path, tee, run, yellow, apple, fish, rain, pen, water, smile, talk, life, sky.

* If above does not help to stop the thoughts about eating just turn your attention away from the invading thoughts about eating. The best way to turn your attention away from the invading thoughts about eating in your head is by doing one of your favorite occupations. Do not be ashamed of any occupation to turn your attention away from the invading thoughts in your head. ALWAYS be busy with your favorite occupation when unsupportable thoughts come to your head.

* Be careful to keep for yourself these of your believes which are found to be strange by the people.

* CONTROL what you say. Say only things which are not strange for the people. You surely already know which of your believes are found to be strange by the people.

* If you do not know yet which of your believes are found to be strange by the people, OBSERVE how people react on what you say. If you see that people are ALERTED by your believes, it means your believes are strange. From now on AVOID presenting such believes.

* Think of three different words, any words which just come to your mind at the moment and make a simple story using these 3 words. Repeat 3 times.

* Try to concentrate on an object close to you, any object. What do you feel when looking at the object? What thoughts come to your mind when looking at the object? And why? Maybe there is a reason. Look for the reason but not too long. If you don't find the reason, forget it.

* Small physical excercise (10 min)

* Small breakfast.

* Nice talk (no complaints, no problematic questions) 10 min. When nobody to talk with, phone or internet conversation oral or written.

* Walk 15 min.

* If you have invading thoughts about eating, ask yourself if it is possible to ignore them.

Yes

Great! In such a case continue ignoring them.

No

You have to learn to ignore the invading thoughts about eating.

This Guide will teach you to ignore the invading thoughts about eating.

Remember: even if you cannot stop the invading thoughts, the invading thoughts cannot stop you to live a normal life.

If you believe in things which other people consider strange, try to keep your strange believes for yourself. Everybody has to make the selection of what can be told to other people and what must be private. Believe me, many people have strange believes. Even much stranger than yours. And they are not considered to be sick. Why? Because they keep their strange believes for themselves. That is the secret.

***

Afternoon

* Say slowly whenever you are invaded by the thoughts about eating: sun, flower, seven, path, tee, run, yellow, apple, fish, rain, pen, water, smile, talk, life, sky.

* Think of three different words, any words which just come to your mind at the moment and make a simple story using these 3 words. Repeat 3 times.

* Try to concentrate on an object close to you, any object. What do you feel when looking at the object? What thoughts come to your mind when looking at the object? And why? Maybe there is a reason. Look for the reason but not too long. If you don't find the reason, forget it.

* Dinner and half an hour break (you can sleep).

* Nice talk (no complaints) 15 min. When nobody to talk with, phone or internet conversation oral or written.

* Walk 20 min.

* If you have the invading thoughts about eating, ask yourself if it is possible to ignore them.

Yes

Great! In such a case continue ignoring them.

No

You have to learn to ignore the invading thoughts.

This Guide will teach you to ignore the invading thoughts about eating.

Remember: even if you cannot stop the invading thoughts, the invading thoughts cannot stop you to live a normal life.

If you believe in things which other people consider strange, try to keep your strange believes for yourself. Everybody has to make the selection of what can be told to other people and what must be private. Believe me, many people have strange believes. Even much stranger than yours. And they are not considered to be sick. Why? Because they keep their strange believes for themselves. That is the secret.

***

Evening

- Say slowly whenever you are invaded by the thoughts about eating: sun, flower, seven, path, tee, run, yellow, apple, fish, rain, pen, water, smile, talk, life, sky.

- Think of three different words, any words which just come to your mind at the moment and make a simple story using these 3 words. Repeat 3 times.

- Try to concentrate on an object close to you, any object. What do you feel when looking at the object? What thoughts come to your mind when looking at the object? And why? Maybe there is a reason. Look for the reason but not too long. If you don't find the reason, forget it.
- Small supper.
- Nice talk (no complaints) 10 min. When nobody to talk with, phone or internet conversation oral or written.
- Walk 10 min.
- If you have the invading thoughts about eating, ask yourself if it is possible to ignore them.

Yes

Great! In such a case continue ignoring them.

No

You have to learn to ignore the invading thoughts.

This Guide will teach you to ignore the invading thoughts.

Remember: even if you cannot stop the invading thoughts, the invading thoughts cannot stop you to live a normal life.

If you believe in things which other people consider strange, try to keep your strange believes for yourself. Everybody has to make the selection of what can be told to other people and what must be private. Believe me, many people have strange believes. Even much stranger than yours. And they are not considered to be sick. Why? Because they keep their strange believes for themselves. That is the secret.

***

Night

Before sleep

- Take a shower (warm water) 1 min.
- Small physical excercise 3 min.

In Bed

- Repeat STOP (10 times if you have invading thoughts).
- Say slowly whenever you are invaded by the thoughts about eating: sun, flower, seven, path, tee, run, yellow, apple, fish, rain, pen, water, smile, talk, life, sky.
- Think of three different words, any words which just come to your mind at the moment and make a simple story using these 3 words. Repeat untill you fall asleep.

If you cannot fall asleep

- Say slowly whenever you are invaded by the thoughts about eating: sun, flower, seven, path, tee, run, yellow, apple, fish, rain, pen, water, smile, talk, life, sky.

If you cannot asleep

- Think of three different words, any words which just come to your mind at the moment and make a simple story using these 3 words. Repeat untill you fall asleep.

If above does not help

- Stand up and go to the toilet (when possible with as little light as possible)
- Say slowly whenever you are invaded by the thoughts about eating: sun, flower, seven, path, tee, run, yellow, apple, fish, rain, pen, water, smile, talk, life, sky.
- Think of three different words, any words which just come to your mind at the moment and make a simple story using these 3 words. Repeat untill you fall asleep.

If above does not help

- Say STOP untill you fall asleep

If above does not help

- Go to the kitchen and have a very small snack.
- Back to the bed think of three different words, any words which just come to your mind at the moment and make a simple story using these 3 words. Repeat untill you fall asleep.
- If above does not help think of three different words, any words which just come to your mind at the moment and make a simple story using these 3 words. Repeat untill you fall asleep.
- Say slowly whenever you are invaded by the thoughts about eating: sun, flower, seven, path, tee, run, yellow, apple, fish, rain, pen, water, smile, talk, life, sky. Repeat untill you fall asleep.

***

Day 2

Morning

* Say STOP whenever thoughts about eating come to your mind.

* Say slowly whenever you are invaded by the thoughts about eating: sun, flower, seven, path, tee, run, yellow, apple, fish, rain, pen, water, smile, talk, life, sky.

* If above does not help to stop the thoughts about eating just turn your attention away from the invading thoughts about eating. The best way to turn your attention away from the invading thoughts about eating in your head is by doing one of your favorite occupations. Do not be ashamed of any occupation to turn your attention away from the invading thoughts in your head. ALWAYS be busy with your favorite occupation when unsupportable thoughts come to your head.

* Be careful to keep for yourself these of your believes which are found to be strange by the people.

* CONTROL what you say. Say only things which are not strange for the people. You surely already know which of your believes are found to be strange by the people.

* If you do not know yet which of your believes are found to be strange by the people, OBSERVE how people react on what you say. If you see that people are ALERTED by your believes, it means your believes are strange. From now on AVOID presenting such believes.

* Think of three different words, any words which just come to your mind at the moment and make a simple story using these 3 words. Repeat 3 times.

* Try to concentrate on an object close to you, any object. What do you feel when looking at the object? What thoughts come to your mind when looking at the object? And why?Maybe there is a reason. Look for the reason but not too long. If you don't find the reason, forget it.

* Small physical excercise (10 min)

* Small breakfast.

* Nice talk (no complaints, no problematic questions) 10 min. When nobody to talk with, phone or internet conversation oral or written.

* Walk 15 min.

* If you have invading thoughts about eating, ask yourself if it is possible to ignore them.

Yes

Great! In such a case continue ignoring them.

No

You have to learn to ignore the invading thoughts about eating.

This Guide will teach you to ignore the invading thoughts about eating.

Remember: even if you cannot stop the invading thoughts, the invading thoughts cannot stop you to live a normal life.

If you believe in things which other people consider strange, try to keep your strange believes for yourself. Everybody has to make the selection of what can be told to other people and what must be private. Believe me, many people have strange believes. Even much stranger than yours. And they are not considered to be sick. Why? Because they keep their strange believes for themselves. That is the secret.

***

Afternoon

* Say slowly whenever you are invaded by the thoughts about eating: sun, flower, seven, path, tee, run, yellow, apple, fish, rain, pen, water, smile, talk, life, sky.

* Think of three different words, any words which just come to your mind at the moment and make a simple story using these 3 words. Repeat 3 times.

* Try to concentrate on an object close to you, any object. What do you feel when looking at the object? What thoughts come to your mind when looking at the

object? And why? Maybe there is a reason. Look for the reason but not too long. If you don't find the reason, forget it.

* Dinner and half an hour break (you can sleep).

* Nice talk (no complaints) 15 min. When nobody to talk with, phone or internet conversation oral or written.

* Walk 20 min.

* If you have the invading thoughts about eating, ask yourself if it is possible to ignore them.

Yes

Great! In such a case continue ignoring them.

No

You have to learn to ignore the invading thoughts.

This Guide will teach you to ignore the invading thoughts about eating.

Remember: even if you cannot stop the invading thoughts, the invading thoughts cannot stop you to live a normal life.

If you believe in things which other people consider strange, try to keep your strange believes for yourself. Everybody has to make the selection of what can be

told to other people and what must be private. Believe me, many people have strange believes. Even much stranger than yours. And they are not considered to be sick. Why? Because they keep their strange believes for themselves. That is the secret.

***

Evening

- Say slowly whenever you are invaded by the thoughts about eating: sun, flower, seven, path, tee, run, yellow, apple, fish, rain, pen, water, smile, talk, life, sky.

- Think of three different words, any words which just come to your mind at the moment and make a simple story using these 3 words. Repeat 3 times.
  - Try to concentrate on an object close to you, any object. What do you feel when looking at the object? What thoughts come to your mind when looking at the object? And why? Maybe there is a reason. Look for the reason but not too long. If you don't find the reason, forget it.
  - Small supper.
  - Nice talk (no complaints) 10 min. When nobody to talk with, phone or internet conversation oral or written.

- Walk 10 min.
- If you have the invading thoughts about eating, ask yourself if it is possible to ignore them.

Yes

Great! In such a case continue ignoring them.

No

You have to learn to ignore the invading thoughts.

This Guide will teach you to ignore the invading thoughts.

Remember: even if you cannot stop the invading thoughts, the invading thoughts cannot stop you to live a normal life.

If you believe in things which other people consider strange, try to keep your strange believes for yourself. Everybody has to make the selection of what can be told to other people and what must be private. Believe me, many people have strange believes. Even much stranger than yours. And they are not considered to be sick. Why? Because they keep their strange believes for themselves. That is the secret.

***

Night

Before sleep

- Take a shower (warm water) 1 min.
- Small physical excercise 3 min.

In Bed

- Repeat STOP (10 times if you have invading thoughts).
- Say slowly whenever you are invaded by the thoughts about eating: sun, flower, seven, path, tee, run, yellow, apple, fish, rain, pen, water, smile, talk, life, sky.
- Think of three different words, any words which just come to your mind at the moment and make a simple story using these 3 words. Repeat untill you fall asleep.

If you cannot fall asleep

- Say slowly whenever you are invaded by the thoughts about eating: sun, flower, seven, path, tee, run, yellow, apple, fish, rain, pen, water, smile, talk, life, sky.

If you cannot asleep

- Think of three different words, any words which just come to your mind at the moment and make a simple story using these 3 words. Repeat untill you fall asleep.

If above does not help

- Stand up and go to the toilet (when possible with as little light as possible)
- Say slowly whenever you are invaded by the thoughts about eating: sun, flower, seven, path, tee, run, yellow, apple, fish, rain, pen, water, smile, talk, life, sky.
- Think of three different words, any words which just come to your mind at the moment and make a simple story using these 3 words. Repeat untill you fall asleep.

If above does not help

- Say STOP untill you fall asleep

If above does not help

- Go to the kitchen and have a very small snack.
- Back to the bed think of three different words, any words which just come to your mind at the moment and make a simple story using these 3 words. Repeat untill you fall asleep.
- If above does not help think of three different words, any words which just come to your mind at the moment and make a simple story using these 3 words. Repeat untill you fall asleep.

- Say slowly whenever you are invaded by the thoughts about eating: sun, flower, seven, path, tee, run, yellow, apple, fish, rain, pen, water, smile, talk, life, sky. Repeat untill you fall asleep.

***

Day 3

Morning

* Say STOP whenever thoughts about eating come to your mind.

* Say slowly whenever you are invaded by the thoughts about eating: sun, flower, seven, path, tee, run, yellow, apple, fish, rain, pen, water, smile, talk, life, sky.

* If above does not help to stop the thoughts about eating just turn your attention away from the invading thoughts about eating. The best way to turn your attention away from the invading thoughts about eating in your head is by doing one of your favorite occupations. Do not be ashamed of any occupation to turn your attention away from the invading thoughts in your head. ALWAYS be busy with your favorite occupation when unsupportable thoughts come to your head.

* Be careful to keep for yourself these of your believes which are found to be strange by the people.

* CONTROL what you say. Say only things which are not strange for the people. You surely already know which of your believes are found to be strange by the people.

* If you do not know yet which of your believes are found to be strange by the people, OBSERVE how people react on what you say. If you see that people are ALERTED by your believes, it means your believes are strange. From now on AVOID presenting such believes.

* Think of three different words, any words which just come to your mind at the moment and make a simple story using these 3 words. Repeat 3 times.

* Try to concentrate on an object close to you, any object. What do you feel when looking at the object? What thoughts come to your mind when looking at the object? And why? Maybe there is a reason. Look for the reason but not too long. If you don't find the reason, forget it.

* Small physical excercise (10 min)

* Small breakfast.

* Nice talk (no complaints, no problematic questions) 10 min. When nobody to talk with, phone or internet conversation oral or written.

* Walk 15 min.

* If you have invading thoughts about eating, ask yourself if it is possible to ignore them.

Yes

Great! In such a case continue ignoring them.

No

You have to learn to ignore the invading thoughts about eating.

This Guide will teach you to ignore the invading thoughts about eating.

Remember: even if you cannot stop the invading thoughts, the invading thoughts cannot stop you to live a normal life.

If you believe in things which other people consider strange, try to keep your strange believes for yourself. Everybody has to make the selection of what can be told to other people and what must be private. Believe me, many people have strange believes. Even much stranger than yours. And they are not considered to be

sick. Why? Because they keep their strange believes for themselves. That is the secret.

***

Afternoon

* Say slowly whenever you are invaded by the thoughts about eating: sun, flower, seven, path, tee, run, yellow, apple, fish, rain, pen, water, smile, talk, life, sky.

* Think of three different words, any words which just come to your mind at the moment and make a simple story using these 3 words. Repeat 3 times.

* Try to concentrate on an object close to you, any object. What do you feel when looking at the object? What thoughts come to your mind when looking at the object? And why? Maybe there is a reason. Look for the reason but not too long. If you don't find the reason, forget it.

* Dinner and half an hour break (you can sleep).

* Nice talk (no complaints) 15 min. When nobody to talk with, phone or internet conversation oral or written.

* Walk 20 min.

* If you have the invading thoughts about eating, ask yourself if it is possible to ignore them.

Yes

Great! In such a case continue ignoring them.

No

You have to learn to ignore the invading thoughts.

This Guide will teach you to ignore the invading thoughts about eating.

Remember: even if you cannot stop the invading thoughts, the invading thoughts cannot stop you to live a normal life.

If you believe in things which other people consider strange, try to keep your strange believes for yourself. Everybody has to make the selection of what can be told to other people and what must be private. Believe me, many people have strange believes. Even much stranger than yours. And they are not considered to be sick. Why? Because they keep their strange believes for themselves. That is the secret.

***

Evening

- Say slowly whenever you are invaded by the thoughts about eating: sun, flower, seven, path, tee, run, yellow, apple, fish, rain, pen, water, smile, talk, life, sky.

- Think of three different words, any words which just come to your mind at the moment and make a simple story using these 3 words. Repeat 3 times.
  - Try to concentrate on an object close to you, any object. What do you feel when looking at the object? What thoughts come to your mind when looking at the object? And why? Maybe there is a reason. Look for the reason but not too long. If you don't find the reason, forget it.
  - Small supper.
  - Nice talk (no complaints) 10 min. When nobody to talk with, phone or internet conversation oral or written.
  - Walk 10 min.
  - If you have the invading thoughts about eating, ask yourself if it is possible to ignore them.

Yes

Great! In such a case continue ignoring them.

No

You have to learn to ignore the invading thoughts.

This Guide will teach you to ignore the invading thoughts.

Remember: even if you cannot stop the invading thoughts, the invading thoughts cannot stop you to live a normal life.

If you believe in things which other people consider strange, try to keep your strange believes for yourself. Everybody has to make the selection of what can be told to other people and what must be private. Believe me, many people have strange believes. Even much stranger than yours. And they are not considered to be sick. Why? Because they keep their strange believes for themselves. That is the secret.

***

Night

Before sleep

- Take a shower (warm water) 1 min.
- Small physical excercise 3 min.

In Bed

- Repeat STOP (10 times if you have invading thoughts).

- Say slowly whenever you are invaded by the thoughts about eating: sun, flower, seven, path, tee, run, yellow, apple, fish, rain, pen, water, smile, talk, life, sky.
- Think of three different words, any words which just come to your mind at the moment and make a simple story using these 3 words. Repeat untill you fall asleep.

If you cannot fall asleep

- Say slowly whenever you are invaded by the thoughts about eating: sun, flower, seven, path, tee, run, yellow, apple, fish, rain, pen, water, smile, talk, life, sky.

If you cannot asleep

- Think of three different words, any words which just come to your mind at the moment and make a simple story using these 3 words. Repeat untill you fall asleep.

If above does not help

- Stand up and go to the toilet (when possible with as little light as possible)
- Say slowly whenever you are invaded by the thoughts about eating: sun, flower, seven, path,

tee, run, yellow, apple, fish, rain, pen, water, smile, talk, life, sky.
- Think of three different words, any words which just come to your mind at the moment and make a simple story using these 3 words. Repeat untill you fall asleep.

If above does not help
- Say STOP untill you fall asleep

If above does not help
- Go to the kitchen and have a very small snack.
- Back to the bed think of three different words, any words which just come to your mind at the moment and make a simple story using these 3 words. Repeat untill you fall asleep.
- If above does not help think of three different words, any words which just come to your mind at the moment and make a simple story using these 3 words. Repeat untill you fall asleep.
- Say slowly whenever you are invaded by the thoughts about eating: sun, flower, seven, path, tee, run, yellow, apple, fish, rain, pen, water, smile, talk, life, sky. Repeat untill you fall asleep.

***

Day 4

Morning

* Say STOP whenever thoughts about eating come to your mind.

* Say slowly whenever you are invaded by the thoughts about eating: sun, flower, seven, path, tee, run, yellow, apple, fish, rain, pen, water, smile, talk, life, sky.

* If above does not help to stop the thoughts about eating just turn your attention away from the invading thoughts about eating. The best way to turn your attention away from the invading thoughts about eating in your head is by doing one of your favorite occupations. Do not be ashamed of any occupation to turn your attention away from the invading thoughts in your head. ALWAYS be busy with your favorite occupation when unsupportable thoughts come to your head.

* Be careful to keep for yourself these of your believes which are found to be strange by the people.

* CONTROL what you say. Say only things which are not strange for the people. You surely already know which of your believes are found to be strange by the people.

* If you do not know yet which of your believes are found to be strange by the people, OBSERVE how

people react on what you say. If you see that people are ALERTED by your believes, it means your believes are strange. From now on AVOID presenting such believes.

* Think of three different words, any words which just come to your mind at the moment and make a simple story using these 3 words. Repeat 3 times.

* Try to concentrate on an object close to you, any object. What do you feel when looking at the object? What thoughts come to your mind when looking at the object? And why? Maybe there is a reason. Look for the reason but not too long. If you don't find the reason, forget it.

* Small physical excercise (10 min)

* Small breakfast.

* Nice talk (no complaints, no problematic questions) 10 min. When nobody to talk with, phone or internet conversation oral or written.

* Walk 15 min.

* If you have invading thoughts about eating, ask yourself if it is possible to ignore them.

Yes

Great! In such a case continue ignoring them.

No

You have to learn to ignore the invading thoughts about eating.

This Guide will teach you to ignore the invading thoughts about eating.

Remember: even if you cannot stop the invading thoughts, the invading thoughts cannot stop you to live a normal life.

If you believe in things which other people consider strange, try to keep your strange believes for yourself. Everybody has to make the selection of what can be told to other people and what must be private. Believe me, many people have strange believes. Even much stranger than yours. And they are not considered to be sick. Why? Because they keep their strange believes for themselves. That is the secret.

***

Afternoon

* Say slowly whenever you are invaded by the thoughts about eating: sun, flower, seven, path, tee, run, yellow, apple, fish, rain, pen, water, smile, talk, life, sky.

* Think of three different words, any words which just come to your mind at the moment and make a simple story using these 3 words. Repeat 3 times.

* Try to concentrate on an object close to you, any object. What do you feel when looking at the object? What thoughts come to your mind when looking at the object? And why? Maybe there is a reason. Look for the reason but not too long. If you don't find the reason, forget it.

* Dinner and half an hour break (you can sleep).

* Nice talk (no complaints) 15 min. When nobody to talk with, phone or internet conversation oral or written.

* Walk 20 min.

* If you have the invading thoughts about eating, ask yourself if it is possible to ignore them.

Yes

Great! In such a case continue ignoring them.

No

You have to learn to ignore the invading thoughts.

This Guide will teach you to ignore the invading thoughts about eating.

Remember: even if you cannot stop the invading thoughts, the invading thoughts cannot stop you to live a normal life.

If you believe in things which other people consider strange, try to keep your strange believes for yourself. Everybody has to make the selection of what can be told to other people and what must be private. Believe me, many people have strange believes. Even much stranger than yours. And they are not considered to be sick. Why? Because they keep their strange believes for themselves. That is the secret.

***

Evening

- Say slowly whenever you are invaded by the thoughts about eating: sun, flower, seven, path, tee, run, yellow, apple, fish, rain, pen, water, smile, talk, life, sky.

- Think of three different words, any words which just come to your mind at the moment and make a simple story using these 3 words. Repeat 3 times.
  - Try to concentrate on an object close to you, any object. What do you feel when looking at the object? What thoughts come to your mind when

looking at the object? And why? Maybe there is a reason. Look for the reason but not too long. If you don't find the reason, forget it.
- Small supper.
- Nice talk (no complaints) 10 min. When nobody to talk with, phone or internet conversation oral or written.
- Walk 10 min.
- If you have the invading thoughts about eating, ask yourself if it is possible to ignore them.

Yes

Great! In such a case continue ignoring them.

No

You have to learn to ignore the invading thoughts.

This Guide will teach you to ignore the invading thoughts.

Remember: even if you cannot stop the invading thoughts, the invading thoughts cannot stop you to live a normal life.

If you believe in things which other people consider strange, try to keep your strange believes for yourself. Everybody has to make the selection of what can be told to other people and what must be private. Believe

me, many people have strange believes. Even much stranger than yours. And they are not considered to be sick. Why? Because they keep their strange believes for themselves. That is the secret.

***

Night

Before sleep

- Take a shower (warm water) 1 min.
- Small physical excercise 3 min.

In Bed

- Repeat STOP (10 times if you have invading thoughts).
- Say slowly whenever you are invaded by the thoughts about eating: sun, flower, seven, path, tee, run, yellow, apple, fish, rain, pen, water, smile, talk, life, sky.
- Think of three different words, any words which just come to your mind at the moment and make a simple story using these 3 words. Repeat untill you fall asleep.

If you cannot fall asleep

- Say slowly whenever you are invaded by the thoughts about eating: sun, flower, seven, path,

tee, run, yellow, apple, fish, rain, pen, water, smile, talk, life, sky.

If you cannot asleep

- Think of three different words, any words which just come to your mind at the moment and make a simple story using these 3 words. Repeat untill you fall asleep.

If above does not help

- Stand up and go to the toilet (when possible with as little light as possible)
- Say slowly whenever you are invaded by the thoughts about eating: sun, flower, seven, path, tee, run, yellow, apple, fish, rain, pen, water, smile, talk, life, sky.
- Think of three different words, any words which just come to your mind at the moment and make a simple story using these 3 words. Repeat untill you fall asleep.

If above does not help

- Say STOP untill you fall asleep

If above does not help

- Go to the kitchen and have a very small snack.

- Back to the bed think of three different words, any words which just come to your mind at the moment and make a simple story using these 3 words. Repeat untill you fall asleep.
- If above does not help think of three different words, any words which just come to your mind at the moment and make a simple story using these 3 words. Repeat untill you fall asleep.
- Say slowly whenever you are invaded by the thoughts about eating: sun, flower, seven, path, tee, run, yellow, apple, fish, rain, pen, water, smile, talk, life, sky. Repeat untill you fall asleep.

***

Day 5

Morning

* Say STOP whenever thoughts about eating come to your mind.

* Say slowly whenever you are invaded by the thoughts about eating: sun, flower, seven, path, tee, run, yellow, apple, fish, rain, pen, water, smile, talk, life, sky.

* If above does not help to stop the thoughts about eating just turn your attention away from the invading thoughts about eating. The best way to turn your

attention away from the invading thoughts about eating in your head is by doing one of your favorite occupations. Do not be ashamed of any occupation to turn your attention away from the invading thoughts in your head. ALWAYS be busy with your favorite occupation when unsupportable thoughts come to your head.

* Be careful to keep for yourself these of your believes which are found to be strange by the people.

* CONTROL what you say. Say only things which are not strange for the people. You surely already know which of your believes are found to be strange by the people.

* If you do not know yet which of your believes are found to be strange by the people, OBSERVE how people react on what you say. If you see that people are ALERTED by your believes, it means your believes are strange. From now on AVOID presenting such believes.

* Think of three different words, any words which just come to your mind at the moment and make a simple story using these 3 words. Repeat 3 times.

* Try to concentrate on an object close to you, any object. What do you feel when looking at the object? What thoughts come to your mind when looking at the object? And why?Maybe there is a reason. Look for the

reason but not too long. If you don't find the reason, forget it.

* Small physical excercise (10 min)

* Small breakfast.

* Nice talk (no complaints, no problematic questions) 10 min. When nobody to talk with, phone or internet conversation oral or written.

* Walk 15 min.

* If you have invading thoughts about eating, ask yourself if it is possible to ignore them.

Yes

Great! In such a case continue ignoring them.

No

You have to learn to ignore the invading thoughts about eating.

This Guide will teach you to ignore the invading thoughts about eating.

Remember: even if you cannot stop the invading thoughts, the invading thoughts cannot stop you to live a normal life.

If you believe in things which other people consider strange, try to keep your strange believes for yourself. Everybody has to make the selection of what can be told to other people and what must be private. Believe me, many people have strange believes. Even much stranger than yours. And they are not considered to be sick. Why? Because they keep their strange believes for themselves. That is the secret.

***

Afternoon

* Say slowly whenever you are invaded by the thoughts about eating: sun, flower, seven, path, tee, run, yellow, apple, fish, rain, pen, water, smile, talk, life, sky.

* Think of three different words, any words which just come to your mind at the moment and make a simple story using these 3 words. Repeat 3 times.

* Try to concentrate on an object close to you, any object. What do you feel when looking at the object? What thoughts come to your mind when looking at the object? And why? Maybe there is a reason. Look for the reason but not too long. If you don't find the reason, forget it.

* Dinner and half an hour break (you can sleep).

* Nice talk (no complaints) 15 min. When nobody to talk with, phone or internet conversation oral or written.

* Walk 20 min.

* If you have the invading thoughts about eating, ask yourself if it is possible to ignore them.

Yes

Great! In such a case continue ignoring them.

No

You have to learn to ignore the invading thoughts.

This Guide will teach you to ignore the invading thoughts about eating.

Remember: even if you cannot stop the invading thoughts, the invading thoughts cannot stop you to live a normal life.

If you believe in things which other people consider strange, try to keep your strange believes for yourself. Everybody has to make the selection of what can be told to other people and what must be private. Believe me, many people have strange believes. Even much stranger than yours. And they are not considered to be

sick. Why? Because they keep their strange believes for themselves. That is the secret.

***

Evening

- Say slowly whenever you are invaded by the thoughts about eating: sun, flower, seven, path, tee, run, yellow, apple, fish, rain, pen, water, smile, talk, life, sky.

- Think of three different words, any words which just come to your mind at the moment and make a simple story using these 3 words. Repeat 3 times.
  - Try to concentrate on an object close to you, any object. What do you feel when looking at the object? What thoughts come to your mind when looking at the object? And why? Maybe there is a reason. Look for the reason but not too long. If you don't find the reason, forget it.
  - Small supper.
  - Nice talk (no complaints) 10 min. When nobody to talk with, phone or internet conversation oral or written.
  - Walk 10 min.
  - If you have the invading thoughts about eating, ask yourself if it is possible to ignore them.

Yes

Great! In such a case continue ignoring them.

No

You have to learn to ignore the invading thoughts.

This Guide will teach you to ignore the invading thoughts.

Remember: even if you cannot stop the invading thoughts, the invading thoughts cannot stop you to live a normal life.

If you believe in things which other people consider strange, try to keep your strange believes for yourself. Everybody has to make the selection of what can be told to other people and what must be private. Believe me, many people have strange believes. Even much stranger than yours. And they are not considered to be sick. Why? Because they keep their strange believes for themselves. That is the secret.

***

Night

Before sleep

- Take a shower (warm water) 1 min.
- Small physical excercise 3 min.

In Bed

- Repeat STOP (10 times if you have invading thoughts).
- Say slowly whenever you are invaded by the thoughts about eating: sun, flower, seven, path, tee, run, yellow, apple, fish, rain, pen, water, smile, talk, life, sky.
- Think of three different words, any words which just come to your mind at the moment and make a simple story using these 3 words. Repeat untill you fall asleep.

If you cannot fall asleep

- Say slowly whenever you are invaded by the thoughts about eating: sun, flower, seven, path, tee, run, yellow, apple, fish, rain, pen, water, smile, talk, life, sky.

If you cannot asleep

- Think of three different words, any words which just come to your mind at the moment and make a simple story using these 3 words. Repeat untill you fall asleep.

If above does not help

- Stand up and go to the toilet (when possible with as little light as possible)

- Say slowly whenever you are invaded by the thoughts about eating: sun, flower, seven, path, tee, run, yellow, apple, fish, rain, pen, water, smile, talk, life, sky.
- Think of three different words, any words which just come to your mind at the moment and make a simple story using these 3 words. Repeat untill you fall asleep.

If above does not help

- Say STOP untill you fall asleep

If above does not help

- Go to the kitchen and have a very small snack.
- Back to the bed think of three different words, any words which just come to your mind at the moment and make a simple story using these 3 words. Repeat untill you fall asleep.
- If above does not help think of three different words, any words which just come to your mind at the moment and make a simple story using these 3 words. Repeat untill you fall asleep.
- Say slowly whenever you are invaded by the thoughts about eating: sun, flower, seven, path, tee, run, yellow, apple, fish, rain, pen, water, smile, talk, life, sky. Repeat untill you fall asleep.

***

Day 6

Morning

* Say STOP whenever thoughts about eating come to your mind.

* Say slowly whenever you are invaded by the thoughts about eating: sun, flower, seven, path, tee, run, yellow, apple, fish, rain, pen, water, smile, talk, life, sky.

* If above does not help to stop the thoughts about eating just turn your attention away from the invading thoughts about eating. The best way to turn your attention away from the invading thoughts about eating in your head is by doing one of your favorite occupations. Do not be ashamed of any occupation to turn your attention away from the invading thoughts in your head. ALWAYS be busy with your favorite occupation when unsupportable thoughts come to your head.

* Be careful to keep for yourself these of your believes which are found to be strange by the people.

* CONTROL what you say. Say only things which are not strange for the people. You surely already know which of your believes are found to be strange by the people.

* If you do not know yet which of your believes are found to be strange by the people, OBSERVE how people react on what you say. If you see that people are ALERTED by your believes, it means your believes are strange. From now on AVOID presenting such believes.

* Think of three different words, any words which just come to your mind at the moment and make a simple story using these 3 words. Repeat 3 times.

* Try to concentrate on an object close to you, any object. What do you feel when looking at the object? What thoughts come to your mind when looking at the object? And why? Maybe there is a reason. Look for the reason but not too long. If you don't find the reason, forget it.

* Small physical excercise (10 min)

* Small breakfast.

* Nice talk (no complaints, no problematic questions) 10 min. When nobody to talk with, phone or internet conversation oral or written.

* Walk 15 min.

* If you have invading thoughts about eating, ask yourself if it is possible to ignore them.

Yes

Great! In such a case continue ignoring them.

No

You have to learn to ignore the invading thoughts about eating.

This Guide will teach you to ignore the invading thoughts about eating.

Remember: even if you cannot stop the invading thoughts, the invading thoughts cannot stop you to live a normal life.

If you believe in things which other people consider strange, try to keep your strange believes for yourself. Everybody has to make the selection of what can be told to other people and what must be private. Believe me, many people have strange believes. Even much stranger than yours. And they are not considered to be sick. Why? Because they keep their strange believes for themselves. That is the secret.

***

Afternoon

* Say slowly whenever you are invaded by the thoughts about eating: sun, flower, seven, path, tee, run, yellow, apple, fish, rain, pen, water, smile, talk, life, sky.

* Think of three different words, any words which just come to your mind at the moment and make a simple story using these 3 words. Repeat 3 times.

* Try to concentrate on an object close to you, any object. What do you feel when looking at the object? What thoughts come to your mind when looking at the object? And why?Maybe there is a reason. Look for the reason but not too long. If you don't find the reason, forget it.

* Dinner and half an hour break (you can sleep).

* Nice talk (no complaints) 15 min. When nobody to talk with, phone or internet conversation oral or written.

* Walk 20 min.

* If you have the invading thoughts about eating, ask yourself if it is possible to ignore them.

Yes

Great! In such a case continue ignoring them.

No

You have to learn to ignore the invading thoughts.

This Guide will teach you to ignore the invading thoughts about eating.

Remember: even if you cannot stop the invading thoughts, the invading thoughts cannot stop you to live a normal life.

If you believe in things which other people consider strange, try to keep your strange believes for yourself. Everybody has to make the selection of what can be told to other people and what must be private. Believe me, many people have strange believes. Even much stranger than yours. And they are not considered to be sick. Why? Because they keep their strange believes for themselves. That is the secret.

***

Evening

- Say slowly whenever you are invaded by the thoughts about eating: sun, flower, seven, path, tee, run, yellow, apple, fish, rain, pen, water, smile, talk, life, sky.

- Think of three different words, any words which just come to your mind at the moment and make a simple story using these 3 words. Repeat 3 times.

- Try to concentrate on an object close to you, any object. What do you feel when looking at the object? What thoughts come to your mind when looking at the object? And why? Maybe there is a reason. Look for the reason but not too long. If you don't find the reason, forget it.
- Small supper.
- Nice talk (no complaints) 10 min. When nobody to talk with, phone or internet conversation oral or written.
- Walk 10 min.
- If you have the invading thoughts about eating, ask yourself if it is possible to ignore them.

Yes

Great! In such a case continue ignoring them.

No

You have to learn to ignore the invading thoughts.

This Guide will teach you to ignore the invading thoughts.

Remember: even if you cannot stop the invading thoughts, the invading thoughts cannot stop you to live a normal life.

If you believe in things which other people consider strange, try to keep your strange believes for yourself. Everybody has to make the selection of what can be told to other people and what must be private. Believe me, many people have strange believes. Even much stranger than yours. And they are not considered to be sick. Why? Because they keep their strange believes for themselves. That is the secret.

***

Night

Before sleep

- Take a shower (warm water) 1 min.
- Small physical excercise 3 min.

In Bed

- Repeat STOP (10 times if you have invading thoughts).
- Say slowly whenever you are invaded by the thoughts about eating: sun, flower, seven, path, tee, run, yellow, apple, fish, rain, pen, water, smile, talk, life, sky.
- Think of three different words, any words which just come to your mind at the moment and make a simple story using these 3 words. Repeat untill you fall asleep.

If you cannot fall asleep

- Say slowly whenever you are invaded by the thoughts about eating: sun, flower, seven, path, tee, run, yellow, apple, fish, rain, pen, water, smile, talk, life, sky.

If you cannot asleep

- Think of three different words, any words which just come to your mind at the moment and make a simple story using these 3 words. Repeat untill you fall asleep.

If above does not help

- Stand up and go to the toilet (when possible with as little light as possible)
- Say slowly whenever you are invaded by the thoughts about eating: sun, flower, seven, path, tee, run, yellow, apple, fish, rain, pen, water, smile, talk, life, sky.
- Think of three different words, any words which just come to your mind at the moment and make a simple story using these 3 words. Repeat untill you fall asleep.

If above does not help

- Say STOP untill you fall asleep

If above does not help

- Go to the kitchen and have a very small snack.
- Back to the bed think of three different words, any words which just come to your mind at the moment and make a simple story using these 3 words. Repeat untill you fall asleep.
- If above does not help think of three different words, any words which just come to your mind at the moment and make a simple story using these 3 words. Repeat untill you fall asleep.
- Say slowly whenever you are invaded by the thoughts about eating: sun, flower, seven, path, tee, run, yellow, apple, fish, rain, pen, water, smile, talk, life, sky. Repeat untill you fall asleep.

***

Day 7

Morning

* Say STOP whenever thoughts about eating come to your mind.

* Say slowly whenever you are invaded by the thoughts about eating: sun, flower, seven, path, tee, run, yellow, apple, fish, rain, pen, water, smile, talk, life, sky.

* If above does not help to stop the thoughts about eating just turn your attention away from the invading thoughts about eating. The best way to turn your attention away from the invading thoughts about eating in your head is by doing one of your favorite occupations. Do not be ashamed of any occupation to turn your attention away from the invading thoughts in your head. ALWAYS be busy with your favorite occupation when unsupportable thoughts come to your head.

* Be careful to keep for yourself these of your believes which are found to be strange by the people.

* CONTROL what you say. Say only things which are not strange for the people. You surely already know which of your believes are found to be strange by the people.

* If you do not know yet which of your believes are found to be strange by the people, OBSERVE how people react on what you say. If you see that people are ALERTED by your believes, it means your believes are strange. From now on AVOID presenting such believes.

* Think of three different words, any words which just come to your mind at the moment and make a simple story using these 3 words. Repeat 3 times.

* Try to concentrate on an object close to you, any object. What do you feel when looking at the object? What thoughts come to your mind when looking at the object? And why?Maybe there is a reason. Look for the reason but not too long. If you don't find the reason, forget it.

* Small physical excercise (10 min)

* Small breakfast.

* Nice talk (no complaints, no problematic questions) 10 min. When nobody to talk with, phone or internet conversation oral or written.

* Walk 15 min.

* If you have invading thoughts about eating, ask yourself if it is possible to ignore them.

Yes

Great! In such a case continue ignoring them.

No

You have to learn to ignore the invading thoughts about eating.

This Guide will teach you to ignore the invading thoughts about eating.

Remember: even if you cannot stop the invading thoughts, the invading thoughts cannot stop you to live a normal life.

If you believe in things which other people consider strange, try to keep your strange believes for yourself. Everybody has to make the selection of what can be told to other people and what must be private. Believe me, many people have strange believes. Even much stranger than yours. And they are not considered to be sick. Why? Because they keep their strange believes for themselves. That is the secret.

***

Afternoon

* Say slowly whenever you are invaded by the thoughts about eating: sun, flower, seven, path, tee, run, yellow, apple, fish, rain, pen, water, smile, talk, life, sky.

* Think of three different words, any words which just come to your mind at the moment and make a simple story using these 3 words. Repeat 3 times.

* Try to concentrate on an object close to you, any object. What do you feel when looking at the object? What thoughts come to your mind when looking at the

object? And why? Maybe there is a reason. Look for the reason but not too long. If you don't find the reason, forget it.

* Dinner and half an hour break (you can sleep).

* Nice talk (no complaints) 15 min. When nobody to talk with, phone or internet conversation oral or written.

* Walk 20 min.

* If you have the invading thoughts about eating, ask yourself if it is possible to ignore them.

Yes

Great! In such a case continue ignoring them.

No

You have to learn to ignore the invading thoughts.

This Guide will teach you to ignore the invading thoughts about eating.

Remember: even if you cannot stop the invading thoughts, the invading thoughts cannot stop you to live a normal life.

If you believe in things which other people consider strange, try to keep your strange believes for yourself. Everybody has to make the selection of what can be

told to other people and what must be private. Believe me, many people have strange believes. Even much stranger than yours. And they are not considered to be sick. Why? Because they keep their strange believes for themselves. That is the secret.

***

Evening

- Say slowly whenever you are invaded by the thoughts about eating: sun, flower, seven, path, tee, run, yellow, apple, fish, rain, pen, water, smile, talk, life, sky.

- Think of three different words, any words which just come to your mind at the moment and make a simple story using these 3 words. Repeat 3 times.
  - Try to concentrate on an object close to you, any object. What do you feel when looking at the object? What thoughts come to your mind when looking at the object? And why? Maybe there is a reason. Look for the reason but not too long. If you don't find the reason, forget it.
  - Small supper.
  - Nice talk (no complaints) 10 min. When nobody to talk with, phone or internet conversation oral or written.

- Walk 10 min.
- If you have the invading thoughts about eating, ask yourself if it is possible to ignore them.

Yes

Great! In such a case continue ignoring them.

No

You have to learn to ignore the invading thoughts.

This Guide will teach you to ignore the invading thoughts.

Remember: even if you cannot stop the invading thoughts, the invading thoughts cannot stop you to live a normal life.

If you believe in things which other people consider strange, try to keep your strange believes for yourself. Everybody has to make the selection of what can be told to other people and what must be private. Believe me, many people have strange believes. Even much stranger than yours. And they are not considered to be sick. Why? Because they keep their strange believes for themselves. That is the secret.

***

Night

Before sleep

- Take a shower (warm water) 1 min.
- Small physical excercise 3 min.

In Bed

- Repeat STOP (10 times if you have invading thoughts).
- Say slowly whenever you are invaded by the thoughts about eating: sun, flower, seven, path, tee, run, yellow, apple, fish, rain, pen, water, smile, talk, life, sky.
- Think of three different words, any words which just come to your mind at the moment and make a simple story using these 3 words. Repeat untill you fall asleep.

If you cannot fall asleep

- Say slowly whenever you are invaded by the thoughts about eating: sun, flower, seven, path, tee, run, yellow, apple, fish, rain, pen, water, smile, talk, life, sky.

If you cannot asleep

- Think of three different words, any words which just come to your mind at the moment and make a simple story using these 3 words. Repeat untill you fall asleep.

If above does not help

- Stand up and go to the toilet (when possible with as little light as possible)
- Say slowly whenever you are invaded by the thoughts about eating: sun, flower, seven, path, tee, run, yellow, apple, fish, rain, pen, water, smile, talk, life, sky.
- Think of three different words, any words which just come to your mind at the moment and make a simple story using these 3 words. Repeat untill you fall asleep.

If above does not help

- Say STOP untill you fall asleep

If above does not help

- Go to the kitchen and have a very small snack.
- Back to the bed think of three different words, any words which just come to your mind at the moment and make a simple story using these 3 words. Repeat untill you fall asleep.
- If above does not help think of three different words, any words which just come to your mind at the moment and make a simple story using these 3 words. Repeat untill you fall asleep.

- Say slowly whenever you are invaded by the thoughts about eating: sun, flower, seven, path, tee, run, yellow, apple, fish, rain, pen, water, smile, talk, life, sky. Repeat untill you fall asleep.

***

Week Four

***

Day 1

Morning

* Say STOP whenever thoughts about eating come to your mind.

* Say slowly whenever you are invaded by the thoughts about eating: sun, flower, seven, path, tee, run, yellow, apple, fish, rain, pen, water, smile, talk, life, sky.

* If above does not help to stop the thoughts about eating just turn your attention away from the invading thoughts about eating. The best way to turn your attention away from the invading thoughts about eating in your head is by doing one of your favorite occupations. Do not be ashamed of any occupation to turn your attention away from the invading thoughts in your head. ALWAYS be busy with your favorite

occupation when unsupportable thoughts come to your head.

* Be careful to keep for yourself these of your believes which are found to be strange by the people.

* CONTROL what you say. Say only things which are not strange for the people. You surely already know which of your believes are found to be strange by the people.

* If you do not know yet which of your believes are found to be strange by the people, OBSERVE how people react on what you say. If you see that people are ALERTED by your believes, it means your believes are strange. From now on AVOID presenting such believes.

* Think of three different words, any words which just come to your mind at the moment and make a simple story using these 3 words. Repeat 3 times.

* Try to concentrate on an object close to you, any object. What do you feel when looking at the object? What thoughts come to your mind when looking at the object? And why?Maybe there is a reason. Look for the reason but not too long. If you don't find the reason, forget it.

* Small physical excercise (10 min)

* Small breakfast.

* Nice talk (no complaints, no problematic questions) 10 min. When nobody to talk with, phone or internet conversation oral or written.

* Walk 15 min.

* If you have invading thoughts about eating, ask yourself if it is possible to ignore them.

Yes

Great! In such a case continue ignoring them.

No

You have to learn to ignore the invading thoughts about eating.

This Guide will teach you to ignore the invading thoughts about eating.

Remember: even if you cannot stop the invading thoughts, the invading thoughts cannot stop you to live a normal life.

If you believe in things which other people consider strange, try to keep your strange believes for yourself. Everybody has to make the selection of what can be told to other people and what must be private. Believe me, many people have strange believes. Even much stranger than yours. And they are not considered to be

sick. Why? Because they keep their strange believes for themselves. That is the secret.

***

Afternoon

* Say slowly whenever you are invaded by the thoughts about eating: sun, flower, seven, path, tee, run, yellow, apple, fish, rain, pen, water, smile, talk, life, sky.

* Think of three different words, any words which just come to your mind at the moment and make a simple story using these 3 words. Repeat 3 times.

* Try to concentrate on an object close to you, any object. What do you feel when looking at the object? What thoughts come to your mind when looking at the object? And why? Maybe there is a reason. Look for the reason but not too long. If you don't find the reason, forget it.

* Dinner and half an hour break (you can sleep).

* Nice talk (no complaints) 15 min. When nobody to talk with, phone or internet conversation oral or written.

* Walk 20 min.

* If you have the invading thoughts about eating, ask yourself if it is possible to ignore them.

Yes

Great! In such a case continue ignoring them.

No

You have to learn to ignore the invading thoughts.

This Guide will teach you to ignore the invading thoughts about eating.

Remember: even if you cannot stop the invading thoughts, the invading thoughts cannot stop you to live a normal life.

If you believe in things which other people consider strange, try to keep your strange believes for yourself. Everybody has to make the selection of what can be told to other people and what must be private. Believe me, many people have strange believes. Even much stranger than yours. And they are not considered to be sick. Why? Because they keep their strange believes for themselves. That is the secret.

***

Evening

- Say slowly whenever you are invaded by the thoughts about eating: sun, flower, seven, path, tee, run, yellow, apple, fish, rain, pen, water, smile, talk, life, sky.

- Think of three different words, any words which just come to your mind at the moment and make a simple story using these 3 words. Repeat 3 times.
  - Try to concentrate on an object close to you, any object. What do you feel when looking at the object? What thoughts come to your mind when looking at the object? And why? Maybe there is a reason. Look for the reason but not too long. If you don't find the reason, forget it.
  - Small supper.
  - Nice talk (no complaints) 10 min. When nobody to talk with, phone or internet conversation oral or written.
  - Walk 10 min.
  - If you have the invading thoughts about eating, ask yourself if it is possible to ignore them.

Yes

Great! In such a case continue ignoring them.

No

You have to learn to ignore the invading thoughts.

This Guide will teach you to ignore the invading thoughts.

Remember: even if you cannot stop the invading thoughts, the invading thoughts cannot stop you to live a normal life.

If you believe in things which other people consider strange, try to keep your strange believes for yourself. Everybody has to make the selection of what can be told to other people and what must be private. Believe me, many people have strange believes. Even much stranger than yours. And they are not considered to be sick. Why? Because they keep their strange believes for themselves. That is the secret.

***

Night

Before sleep

- Take a shower (warm water) 1 min.
- Small physical excercise 3 min.

In Bed

- Repeat STOP (10 times if you have invading thoughts).

- Say slowly whenever you are invaded by the thoughts about eating: sun, flower, seven, path, tee, run, yellow, apple, fish, rain, pen, water, smile, talk, life, sky.
- Think of three different words, any words which just come to your mind at the moment and make a simple story using these 3 words. Repeat untill you fall asleep.

If you cannot fall asleep

- Say slowly whenever you are invaded by the thoughts about eating: sun, flower, seven, path, tee, run, yellow, apple, fish, rain, pen, water, smile, talk, life, sky.

If you cannot asleep

- Think of three different words, any words which just come to your mind at the moment and make a simple story using these 3 words. Repeat untill you fall asleep.

If above does not help

- Stand up and go to the toilet (when possible with as little light as possible)
- Say slowly whenever you are invaded by the thoughts about eating: sun, flower, seven, path,

tee, run, yellow, apple, fish, rain, pen, water, smile, talk, life, sky.
- Think of three different words, any words which just come to your mind at the moment and make a simple story using these 3 words. Repeat untill you fall asleep.

If above does not help
- Say STOP untill you fall asleep

If above does not help

- Go to the kitchen and have a very small snack.
- Back to the bed think of three different words, any words which just come to your mind at the moment and make a simple story using these 3 words. Repeat untill you fall asleep.
- If above does not help think of three different words, any words which just come to your mind at the moment and make a simple story using these 3 words. Repeat untill you fall asleep.
- Say slowly whenever you are invaded by the thoughts about eating: sun, flower, seven, path, tee, run, yellow, apple, fish, rain, pen, water, smile, talk, life, sky. Repeat untill you fall asleep.

***

Day 2

Morning

* Say STOP whenever thoughts about eating come to your mind.

* Say slowly whenever you are invaded by the thoughts about eating: sun, flower, seven, path, tee, run, yellow, apple, fish, rain, pen, water, smile, talk, life, sky.

* If above does not help to stop the thoughts about eating just turn your attention away from the invading thoughts about eating. The best way to turn your attention away from the invading thoughts about eating in your head is by doing one of your favorite occupations. Do not be ashamed of any occupation to turn your attention away from the invading thoughts in your head. ALWAYS be busy with your favorite occupation when unsupportable thoughts come to your head.

* Be careful to keep for yourself these of your believes which are found to be strange by the people.

* CONTROL what you say. Say only things which are not strange for the people. You surely already know which of your believes are found to be strange by the people.

* If you do not know yet which of your believes are found to be strange by the people, OBSERVE how

people react on what you say. If you see that people are ALERTED by your believes, it means your believes are strange. From now on AVOID presenting such believes.

* Think of three different words, any words which just come to your mind at the moment and make a simple story using these 3 words. Repeat 3 times.

* Try to concentrate on an object close to you, any object. What do you feel when looking at the object? What thoughts come to your mind when looking at the object? And why? Maybe there is a reason. Look for the reason but not too long. If you don't find the reason, forget it.

* Small physical excercise (10 min)

* Small breakfast.

* Nice talk (no complaints, no problematic questions) 10 min. When nobody to talk with, phone or internet conversation oral or written.

* Walk 15 min.

* If you have invading thoughts about eating, ask yourself if it is possible to ignore them.

Yes

Great! In such a case continue ignoring them.

No

You have to learn to ignore the invading thoughts about eating.

This Guide will teach you to ignore the invading thoughts about eating.

Remember: even if you cannot stop the invading thoughts, the invading thoughts cannot stop you to live a normal life.

If you believe in things which other people consider strange, try to keep your strange believes for yourself. Everybody has to make the selection of what can be told to other people and what must be private. Believe me, many people have strange believes. Even much stranger than yours. And they are not considered to be sick. Why? Because they keep their strange believes for themselves. That is the secret.

***

Afternoon

* Say slowly whenever you are invaded by the thoughts about eating: sun, flower, seven, path, tee, run, yellow, apple, fish, rain, pen, water, smile, talk, life, sky.

* Think of three different words, any words which just come to your mind at the moment and make a simple story using these 3 words. Repeat 3 times.

* Try to concentrate on an object close to you, any object. What do you feel when looking at the object? What thoughts come to your mind when looking at the object? And why? Maybe there is a reason. Look for the reason but not too long. If you don't find the reason, forget it.

* Dinner and half an hour break (you can sleep).

* Nice talk (no complaints) 15 min. When nobody to talk with, phone or internet conversation oral or written.

* Walk 20 min.

* If you have the invading thoughts about eating, ask yourself if it is possible to ignore them.

Yes

Great! In such a case continue ignoring them.

No

You have to learn to ignore the invading thoughts.

This Guide will teach you to ignore the invading thoughts about eating.

Remember: even if you cannot stop the invading thoughts, the invading thoughts cannot stop you to live a normal life.

If you believe in things which other people consider strange, try to keep your strange believes for yourself. Everybody has to make the selection of what can be told to other people and what must be private. Believe me, many people have strange believes. Even much stranger than yours. And they are not considered to be sick. Why? Because they keep their strange believes for themselves. That is the secret.

***

Evening

- Say slowly whenever you are invaded by the thoughts about eating: sun, flower, seven, path, tee, run, yellow, apple, fish, rain, pen, water, smile, talk, life, sky.

- Think of three different words, any words which just come to your mind at the moment and make a simple story using these 3 words. Repeat 3 times.
    - Try to concentrate on an object close to you, any object. What do you feel when looking at the object? What thoughts come to your mind when

looking at the object? And why? Maybe there is a reason. Look for the reason but not too long. If you don't find the reason, forget it.

- Small supper.
- Nice talk (no complaints) 10 min. When nobody to talk with, phone or internet conversation oral or written.
- Walk 10 min.
- If you have the invading thoughts about eating, ask yourself if it is possible to ignore them.

Yes

Great! In such a case continue ignoring them.

No

You have to learn to ignore the invading thoughts.

This Guide will teach you to ignore the invading thoughts.

Remember: even if you cannot stop the invading thoughts, the invading thoughts cannot stop you to live a normal life.

If you believe in things which other people consider strange, try to keep your strange believes for yourself. Everybody has to make the selection of what can be told to other people and what must be private. Believe

me, many people have strange believes. Even much stranger than yours. And they are not considered to be sick. Why? Because they keep their strange believes for themselves. That is the secret.

***

Night

Before sleep

- Take a shower (warm water) 1 min.
- Small physical excercise 3 min.

In Bed

- Repeat STOP (10 times if you have invading thoughts).
- Say slowly whenever you are invaded by the thoughts about eating: sun, flower, seven, path, tee, run, yellow, apple, fish, rain, pen, water, smile, talk, life, sky.
- Think of three different words, any words which just come to your mind at the moment and make a simple story using these 3 words. Repeat untill you fall asleep.

If you cannot fall asleep

- Say slowly whenever you are invaded by the thoughts about eating: sun, flower, seven, path,

tee, run, yellow, apple, fish, rain, pen, water, smile, talk, life, sky.

If you cannot asleep

- Think of three different words, any words which just come to your mind at the moment and make a simple story using these 3 words. Repeat untill you fall asleep.

If above does not help

- Stand up and go to the toilet (when possible with as little light as possible)
- Say slowly whenever you are invaded by the thoughts about eating: sun, flower, seven, path, tee, run, yellow, apple, fish, rain, pen, water, smile, talk, life, sky.
- Think of three different words, any words which just come to your mind at the moment and make a simple story using these 3 words. Repeat untill you fall asleep.

If above does not help

- Say STOP untill you fall asleep

If above does not help

- Go to the kitchen and have a very small snack.

- Back to the bed think of three different words, any words which just come to your mind at the moment and make a simple story using these 3 words. Repeat untill you fall asleep.
- If above does not help think of three different words, any words which just come to your mind at the moment and make a simple story using these 3 words. Repeat untill you fall asleep.
- Say slowly whenever you are invaded by the thoughts about eating: sun, flower, seven, path, tee, run, yellow, apple, fish, rain, pen, water, smile, talk, life, sky. Repeat untill you fall asleep.

***

Day 3

Morning

* Say STOP whenever thoughts about eating come to your mind.

* Say slowly whenever you are invaded by the thoughts about eating: sun, flower, seven, path, tee, run, yellow, apple, fish, rain, pen, water, smile, talk, life, sky.

* If above does not help to stop the thoughts about eating just turn your attention away from the invading thoughts about eating. The best way to turn your

attention away from the invading thoughts about eating in your head is by doing one of your favorite occupations. Do not be ashamed of any occupation to turn your attention away from the invading thoughts in your head. ALWAYS be busy with your favorite occupation when unsupportable thoughts come to your head.

* Be careful to keep for yourself these of your believes which are found to be strange by the people.

* CONTROL what you say. Say only things which are not strange for the people. You surely already know which of your believes are found to be strange by the people.

* If you do not know yet which of your believes are found to be strange by the people, OBSERVE how people react on what you say. If you see that people are ALERTED by your believes, it means your believes are strange. From now on AVOID presenting such believes.

* Think of three different words, any words which just come to your mind at the moment and make a simple story using these 3 words. Repeat 3 times.

* Try to concentrate on an object close to you, any object. What do you feel when looking at the object? What thoughts come to your mind when looking at the object? And why?Maybe there is a reason. Look for the

reason but not too long. If you don't find the reason, forget it.

* Small physical excercise (10 min)

* Small breakfast.

* Nice talk (no complaints, no problematic questions) 10 min. When nobody to talk with, phone or internet conversation oral or written.

* Walk 15 min.

* If you have invading thoughts about eating, ask yourself if it is possible to ignore them.

Yes

Great! In such a case continue ignoring them.

No

You have to learn to ignore the invading thoughts about eating.

This Guide will teach you to ignore the invading thoughts about eating.

Remember: even if you cannot stop the invading thoughts, the invading thoughts cannot stop you to live a normal life.

If you believe in things which other people consider strange, try to keep your strange believes for yourself. Everybody has to make the selection of what can be told to other people and what must be private. Believe me, many people have strange believes. Even much stranger than yours. And they are not considered to be sick. Why? Because they keep their strange believes for themselves. That is the secret.

***

Afternoon

* Say slowly whenever you are invaded by the thoughts about eating: sun, flower, seven, path, tee, run, yellow, apple, fish, rain, pen, water, smile, talk, life, sky.

* Think of three different words, any words which just come to your mind at the moment and make a simple story using these 3 words. Repeat 3 times.

* Try to concentrate on an object close to you, any object. What do you feel when looking at the object? What thoughts come to your mind when looking at the object? And why? Maybe there is a reason. Look for the reason but not too long. If you don't find the reason, forget it.

* Dinner and half an hour break (you can sleep).

* Nice talk (no complaints) 15 min. When nobody to talk with, phone or internet conversation oral or written.

* Walk 20 min.

* If you have the invading thoughts about eating, ask yourself if it is possible to ignore them.

Yes

Great! In such a case continue ignoring them.

No

You have to learn to ignore the invading thoughts.

This Guide will teach you to ignore the invading thoughts about eating.

Remember: even if you cannot stop the invading thoughts, the invading thoughts cannot stop you to live a normal life.

If you believe in things which other people consider strange, try to keep your strange believes for yourself. Everybody has to make the selection of what can be told to other people and what must be private. Believe me, many people have strange believes. Even much stranger than yours. And they are not considered to be

sick. Why? Because they keep their strange believes for themselves. That is the secret.

***

Evening

- Say slowly whenever you are invaded by the thoughts about eating: sun, flower, seven, path, tee, run, yellow, apple, fish, rain, pen, water, smile, talk, life, sky.

- Think of three different words, any words which just come to your mind at the moment and make a simple story using these 3 words. Repeat 3 times.
  - Try to concentrate on an object close to you, any object. What do you feel when looking at the object? What thoughts come to your mind when looking at the object? And why? Maybe there is a reason. Look for the reason but not too long. If you don't find the reason, forget it.
  - Small supper.
  - Nice talk (no complaints) 10 min. When nobody to talk with, phone or internet conversation oral or written.
  - Walk 10 min.
  - If you have the invading thoughts about eating, ask yourself if it is possible to ignore them.

Yes

Great! In such a case continue ignoring them.

No

You have to learn to ignore the invading thoughts.

This Guide will teach you to ignore the invading thoughts.

Remember: even if you cannot stop the invading thoughts, the invading thoughts cannot stop you to live a normal life.

If you believe in things which other people consider strange, try to keep your strange believes for yourself. Everybody has to make the selection of what can be told to other people and what must be private. Believe me, many people have strange believes. Even much stranger than yours. And they are not considered to be sick. Why? Because they keep their strange believes for themselves. That is the secret.

***

Night

Before sleep

- Take a shower (warm water) 1 min.
- Small physical excercise 3 min.

In Bed

- Repeat STOP (10 times if you have invading thoughts).
- Say slowly whenever you are invaded by the thoughts about eating: sun, flower, seven, path, tee, run, yellow, apple, fish, rain, pen, water, smile, talk, life, sky.
- Think of three different words, any words which just come to your mind at the moment and make a simple story using these 3 words. Repeat untill you fall asleep.

If you cannot fall asleep

- Say slowly whenever you are invaded by the thoughts about eating: sun, flower, seven, path, tee, run, yellow, apple, fish, rain, pen, water, smile, talk, life, sky.

If you cannot asleep

- Think of three different words, any words which just come to your mind at the moment and make a simple story using these 3 words. Repeat untill you fall asleep.

If above does not help

- Stand up and go to the toilet (when possible with as little light as possible)

- Say slowly whenever you are invaded by the thoughts about eating: sun, flower, seven, path, tee, run, yellow, apple, fish, rain, pen, water, smile, talk, life, sky.
- Think of three different words, any words which just come to your mind at the moment and make a simple story using these 3 words. Repeat untill you fall asleep.

If above does not help

- Say STOP untill you fall asleep

If above does not help

- Go to the kitchen and have a very small snack.
- Back to the bed think of three different words, any words which just come to your mind at the moment and make a simple story using these 3 words. Repeat untill you fall asleep.
- If above does not help think of three different words, any words which just come to your mind at the moment and make a simple story using these 3 words. Repeat untill you fall asleep.
- Say slowly whenever you are invaded by the thoughts about eating: sun, flower, seven, path, tee, run, yellow, apple, fish, rain, pen, water, smile, talk, life, sky. Repeat untill you fall asleep.

***

Day 4

Morning

* Say STOP whenever thoughts about eating come to your mind.

* Say slowly whenever you are invaded by the thoughts about eating: sun, flower, seven, path, tee, run, yellow, apple, fish, rain, pen, water, smile, talk, life, sky.

* If above does not help to stop the thoughts about eating just turn your attention away from the invading thoughts about eating. The best way to turn your attention away from the invading thoughts about eating in your head is by doing one of your favorite occupations. Do not be ashamed of any occupation to turn your attention away from the invading thoughts in your head. ALWAYS be busy with your favorite occupation when unsupportable thoughts come to your head.

* Be careful to keep for yourself these of your believes which are found to be strange by the people.

* CONTROL what you say. Say only things which are not strange for the people. You surely already know which of your believes are found to be strange by the people.

* If you do not know yet which of your believes are found to be strange by the people, OBSERVE how people react on what you say. If you see that people are ALERTED by your believes, it means your believes are strange. From now on AVOID presenting such believes.

* Think of three different words, any words which just come to your mind at the moment and make a simple story using these 3 words. Repeat 3 times.

* Try to concentrate on an object close to you, any object. What do you feel when looking at the object? What thoughts come to your mind when looking at the object? And why? Maybe there is a reason. Look for the reason but not too long. If you don't find the reason, forget it.

* Small physical excercise (10 min)

* Small breakfast.

* Nice talk (no complaints, no problematic questions) 10 min. When nobody to talk with, phone or internet conversation oral or written.

* Walk 15 min.

* If you have invading thoughts about eating, ask yourself if it is possible to ignore them.

Yes

Great! In such a case continue ignoring them.

No

You have to learn to ignore the invading thoughts about eating.

This Guide will teach you to ignore the invading thoughts about eating.

Remember: even if you cannot stop the invading thoughts, the invading thoughts cannot stop you to live a normal life.

If you believe in things which other people consider strange, try to keep your strange believes for yourself. Everybody has to make the selection of what can be told to other people and what must be private. Believe me, many people have strange believes. Even much stranger than yours. And they are not considered to be sick. Why? Because they keep their strange believes for themselves. That is the secret.

***

Afternoon

* Say slowly whenever you are invaded by the thoughts about eating: sun, flower, seven, path, tee, run, yellow, apple, fish, rain, pen, water, smile, talk, life, sky.

* Think of three different words, any words which just come to your mind at the moment and make a simple story using these 3 words. Repeat 3 times.

* Try to concentrate on an object close to you, any object. What do you feel when looking at the object? What thoughts come to your mind when looking at the object? And why? Maybe there is a reason. Look for the reason but not too long. If you don't find the reason, forget it.

* Dinner and half an hour break (you can sleep).

* Nice talk (no complaints) 15 min. When nobody to talk with, phone or internet conversation oral or written.

* Walk 20 min.

* If you have the invading thoughts about eating, ask yourself if it is possible to ignore them.

Yes

Great! In such a case continue ignoring them.

No

You have to learn to ignore the invading thoughts.

This Guide will teach you to ignore the invading thoughts about eating.

Remember: even if you cannot stop the invading thoughts, the invading thoughts cannot stop you to live a normal life.

If you believe in things which other people consider strange, try to keep your strange believes for yourself. Everybody has to make the selection of what can be told to other people and what must be private. Believe me, many people have strange believes. Even much stranger than yours. And they are not considered to be sick. Why? Because they keep their strange believes for themselves. That is the secret.

***

Evening

- Say slowly whenever you are invaded by the thoughts about eating: sun, flower, seven, path, tee, run, yellow, apple, fish, rain, pen, water, smile, talk, life, sky.

- Think of three different words, any words which just come to your mind at the moment and make a simple story using these 3 words. Repeat 3 times.

- Try to concentrate on an object close to you, any object. What do you feel when looking at the object? What thoughts come to your mind when looking at the object? And why? Maybe there is a reason. Look for the reason but not too long. If you don't find the reason, forget it.
- Small supper.
- Nice talk (no complaints) 10 min. When nobody to talk with, phone or internet conversation oral or written.
- Walk 10 min.
- If you have the invading thoughts about eating, ask yourself if it is possible to ignore them.

Yes

Great! In such a case continue ignoring them.

No

You have to learn to ignore the invading thoughts.

This Guide will teach you to ignore the invading thoughts.

Remember: even if you cannot stop the invading thoughts, the invading thoughts cannot stop you to live a normal life.

If you believe in things which other people consider strange, try to keep your strange believes for yourself. Everybody has to make the selection of what can be told to other people and what must be private. Believe me, many people have strange believes. Even much stranger than yours. And they are not considered to be sick. Why? Because they keep their strange believes for themselves. That is the secret.

***

Night

Before sleep

- Take a shower (warm water) 1 min.
- Small physical excercise 3 min.

In Bed

- Repeat STOP (10 times if you have invading thoughts).
- Say slowly whenever you are invaded by the thoughts about eating: sun, flower, seven, path, tee, run, yellow, apple, fish, rain, pen, water, smile, talk, life, sky.
- Think of three different words, any words which just come to your mind at the moment and make a simple story using these 3 words. Repeat untill you fall asleep.

If you cannot fall asleep

- Say slowly whenever you are invaded by the thoughts about eating: sun, flower, seven, path, tee, run, yellow, apple, fish, rain, pen, water, smile, talk, life, sky.

If you cannot asleep

- Think of three different words, any words which just come to your mind at the moment and make a simple story using these 3 words. Repeat untill you fall asleep.

If above does not help

- Stand up and go to the toilet (when possible with as little light as possible)
- Say slowly whenever you are invaded by the thoughts about eating: sun, flower, seven, path, tee, run, yellow, apple, fish, rain, pen, water, smile, talk, life, sky.
- Think of three different words, any words which just come to your mind at the moment and make a simple story using these 3 words. Repeat untill you fall asleep.

If above does not help

- Say STOP untill you fall asleep

If above does not help

- Go to the kitchen and have a very small snack.
- Back to the bed think of three different words, any words which just come to your mind at the moment and make a simple story using these 3 words. Repeat untill you fall asleep.
- If above does not help think of three different words, any words which just come to your mind at the moment and make a simple story using these 3 words. Repeat untill you fall asleep.
- Say slowly whenever you are invaded by the thoughts about eating: sun, flower, seven, path, tee, run, yellow, apple, fish, rain, pen, water, smile, talk, life, sky. Repeat untill you fall asleep.

***

Day 5

Morning

* Say STOP whenever thoughts about eating come to your mind.

* Say slowly whenever you are invaded by the thoughts about eating: sun, flower, seven, path, tee, run, yellow, apple, fish, rain, pen, water, smile, talk, life, sky.

* If above does not help to stop the thoughts about eating just turn your attention away from the invading thoughts about eating. The best way to turn your attention away from the invading thoughts about eating in your head is by doing one of your favorite occupations. Do not be ashamed of any occupation to turn your attention away from the invading thoughts in your head. ALWAYS be busy with your favorite occupation when unsupportable thoughts come to your head.

* Be careful to keep for yourself these of your believes which are found to be strange by the people.

* CONTROL what you say. Say only things which are not strange for the people. You surely already know which of your believes are found to be strange by the people.

* If you do not know yet which of your believes are found to be strange by the people, OBSERVE how people react on what you say. If you see that people are ALERTED by your believes, it means your believes are strange. From now on AVOID presenting such believes.

* Think of three different words, any words which just come to your mind at the moment and make a simple story using these 3 words. Repeat 3 times.

* Try to concentrate on an object close to you, any object. What do you feel when looking at the object? What thoughts come to your mind when looking at the object? And why? Maybe there is a reason. Look for the reason but not too long. If you don't find the reason, forget it.

* Small physical excercise (10 min)

* Small breakfast.

* Nice talk (no complaints, no problematic questions) 10 min. When nobody to talk with, phone or internet conversation oral or written.

* Walk 15 min.

* If you have invading thoughts about eating, ask yourself if it is possible to ignore them.

Yes

Great! In such a case continue ignoring them.

No

You have to learn to ignore the invading thoughts about eating.

This Guide will teach you to ignore the invading thoughts about eating.

Remember: even if you cannot stop the invading thoughts, the invading thoughts cannot stop you to live a normal life.

If you believe in things which other people consider strange, try to keep your strange believes for yourself. Everybody has to make the selection of what can be told to other people and what must be private. Believe me, many people have strange believes. Even much stranger than yours. And they are not considered to be sick. Why? Because they keep their strange believes for themselves. That is the secret.

***

Afternoon

* Say slowly whenever you are invaded by the thoughts about eating: sun, flower, seven, path, tee, run, yellow, apple, fish, rain, pen, water, smile, talk, life, sky.

* Think of three different words, any words which just come to your mind at the moment and make a simple story using these 3 words. Repeat 3 times.

* Try to concentrate on an object close to you, any object. What do you feel when looking at the object? What thoughts come to your mind when looking at the

object? And why? Maybe there is a reason. Look for the reason but not too long. If you don't find the reason, forget it.

* Dinner and half an hour break (you can sleep).

* Nice talk (no complaints) 15 min. When nobody to talk with, phone or internet conversation oral or written.

* Walk 20 min.

* If you have the invading thoughts about eating, ask yourself if it is possible to ignore them.

Yes

Great! In such a case continue ignoring them.

No

You have to learn to ignore the invading thoughts.

This Guide will teach you to ignore the invading thoughts about eating.

Remember: even if you cannot stop the invading thoughts, the invading thoughts cannot stop you to live a normal life.

If you believe in things which other people consider strange, try to keep your strange believes for yourself. Everybody has to make the selection of what can be

told to other people and what must be private. Believe me, many people have strange believes. Even much stranger than yours. And they are not considered to be sick. Why? Because they keep their strange believes for themselves. That is the secret.

***

Evening

- Say slowly whenever you are invaded by the thoughts about eating: sun, flower, seven, path, tee, run, yellow, apple, fish, rain, pen, water, smile, talk, life, sky.

- Think of three different words, any words which just come to your mind at the moment and make a simple story using these 3 words. Repeat 3 times.
  - Try to concentrate on an object close to you, any object. What do you feel when looking at the object? What thoughts come to your mind when looking at the object? And why? Maybe there is a reason. Look for the reason but not too long. If you don't find the reason, forget it.
  - Small supper.
  - Nice talk (no complaints) 10 min. When nobody to talk with, phone or internet conversation oral or written.

- Walk 10 min.
- If you have the invading thoughts about eating, ask yourself if it is possible to ignore them.

Yes

Great! In such a case continue ignoring them.

No

You have to learn to ignore the invading thoughts.

This Guide will teach you to ignore the invading thoughts.

Remember: even if you cannot stop the invading thoughts, the invading thoughts cannot stop you to live a normal life.

If you believe in things which other people consider strange, try to keep your strange believes for yourself. Everybody has to make the selection of what can be told to other people and what must be private. Believe me, many people have strange believes. Even much stranger than yours. And they are not considered to be sick. Why? Because they keep their strange believes for themselves. That is the secret.

***

Night

Before sleep

- Take a shower (warm water) 1 min.
- Small physical excercise 3 min.

In Bed

- Repeat STOP (10 times if you have invading thoughts).
- Say slowly whenever you are invaded by the thoughts about eating: sun, flower, seven, path, tee, run, yellow, apple, fish, rain, pen, water, smile, talk, life, sky.
- Think of three different words, any words which just come to your mind at the moment and make a simple story using these 3 words. Repeat untill you fall asleep.

If you cannot fall asleep

- Say slowly whenever you are invaded by the thoughts about eating: sun, flower, seven, path, tee, run, yellow, apple, fish, rain, pen, water, smile, talk, life, sky.

If you cannot asleep

- Think of three different words, any words which just come to your mind at the moment and make a simple story using these 3 words. Repeat untill you fall asleep.

If above does not help

- Stand up and go to the toilet (when possible with as little light as possible)
- Say slowly whenever you are invaded by the thoughts about eating: sun, flower, seven, path, tee, run, yellow, apple, fish, rain, pen, water, smile, talk, life, sky.
- Think of three different words, any words which just come to your mind at the moment and make a simple story using these 3 words. Repeat untill you fall asleep.

If above does not help

- Say STOP untill you fall asleep

If above does not help

- Go to the kitchen and have a very small snack.
- Back to the bed think of three different words, any words which just come to your mind at the moment and make a simple story using these 3 words. Repeat untill you fall asleep.
- If above does not help think of three different words, any words which just come to your mind at the moment and make a simple story using these 3 words. Repeat untill you fall asleep.

- Say slowly whenever you are invaded by the thoughts about eating: sun, flower, seven, path, tee, run, yellow, apple, fish, rain, pen, water, smile, talk, life, sky. Repeat untill you fall asleep.

***

Day 6

Morning

* Say STOP whenever thoughts about eating come to your mind.

* Say slowly whenever you are invaded by the thoughts about eating: sun, flower, seven, path, tee, run, yellow, apple, fish, rain, pen, water, smile, talk, life, sky.

* If above does not help to stop the thoughts about eating just turn your attention away from the invading thoughts about eating. The best way to turn your attention away from the invading thoughts about eating in your head is by doing one of your favorite occupations. Do not be ashamed of any occupation to turn your attention away from the invading thoughts in your head. ALWAYS be busy with your favorite occupation when unsupportable thoughts come to your head.

* Be careful to keep for yourself these of your believes which are found to be strange by the people.

* CONTROL what you say. Say only things which are not strange for the people. You surely already know which of your believes are found to be strange by the people.

* If you do not know yet which of your believes are found to be strange by the people, OBSERVE how people react on what you say. If you see that people are ALERTED by your believes, it means your believes are strange. From now on AVOID presenting such believes.

* Think of three different words, any words which just come to your mind at the moment and make a simple story using these 3 words. Repeat 3 times.

* Try to concentrate on an object close to you, any object. What do you feel when looking at the object? What thoughts come to your mind when looking at the object? And why? Maybe there is a reason. Look for the reason but not too long. If you don't find the reason, forget it.

* Small physical excercise (10 min)

* Small breakfast.

* Nice talk (no complaints, no problematic questions) 10 min. When nobody to talk with, phone or internet conversation oral or written.

* Walk 15 min.

* If you have invading thoughts about eating, ask yourself if it is possible to ignore them.

Yes

Great! In such a case continue ignoring them.

No

You have to learn to ignore the invading thoughts about eating.

This Guide will teach you to ignore the invading thoughts about eating.

Remember: even if you cannot stop the invading thoughts, the invading thoughts cannot stop you to live a normal life.

If you believe in things which other people consider strange, try to keep your strange believes for yourself. Everybody has to make the selection of what can be told to other people and what must be private. Believe me, many people have strange believes. Even much stranger than yours. And they are not considered to be

sick. Why? Because they keep their strange believes for themselves. That is the secret.

***

Afternoon

* Say slowly whenever you are invaded by the thoughts about eating: sun, flower, seven, path, tee, run, yellow, apple, fish, rain, pen, water, smile, talk, life, sky.

* Think of three different words, any words which just come to your mind at the moment and make a simple story using these 3 words. Repeat 3 times.

* Try to concentrate on an object close to you, any object. What do you feel when looking at the object? What thoughts come to your mind when looking at the object? And why? Maybe there is a reason. Look for the reason but not too long. If you don't find the reason, forget it.

* Dinner and half an hour break (you can sleep).

* Nice talk (no complaints) 15 min. When nobody to talk with, phone or internet conversation oral or written.

* Walk 20 min.

* If you have the invading thoughts about eating, ask yourself if it is possible to ignore them.

Yes

Great! In such a case continue ignoring them.

No

You have to learn to ignore the invading thoughts.

This Guide will teach you to ignore the invading thoughts about eating.

Remember: even if you cannot stop the invading thoughts, the invading thoughts cannot stop you to live a normal life.

If you believe in things which other people consider strange, try to keep your strange believes for yourself. Everybody has to make the selection of what can be told to other people and what must be private. Believe me, many people have strange believes. Even much stranger than yours. And they are not considered to be sick. Why? Because they keep their strange believes for themselves. That is the secret.

***

Evening

- Say slowly whenever you are invaded by the thoughts about eating: sun, flower, seven, path, tee, run, yellow, apple, fish, rain, pen, water, smile, talk, life, sky.

- Think of three different words, any words which just come to your mind at the moment and make a simple story using these 3 words. Repeat 3 times.
  - Try to concentrate on an object close to you, any object. What do you feel when looking at the object? What thoughts come to your mind when looking at the object? And why? Maybe there is a reason. Look for the reason but not too long. If you don't find the reason, forget it.
  - Small supper.
  - Nice talk (no complaints) 10 min. When nobody to talk with, phone or internet conversation oral or written.
  - Walk 10 min.
  - If you have the invading thoughts about eating, ask yourself if it is possible to ignore them.

Yes

Great! In such a case continue ignoring them.

No

You have to learn to ignore the invading thoughts.

This Guide will teach you to ignore the invading thoughts.

Remember: even if you cannot stop the invading thoughts, the invading thoughts cannot stop you to live a normal life.

If you believe in things which other people consider strange, try to keep your strange believes for yourself. Everybody has to make the selection of what can be told to other people and what must be private. Believe me, many people have strange believes. Even much stranger than yours. And they are not considered to be sick. Why? Because they keep their strange believes for themselves. That is the secret.

***

Night

Before sleep

- Take a shower (warm water) 1 min.
- Small physical excercise 3 min.

In Bed

- Repeat STOP (10 times if you have invading thoughts).

- Say slowly whenever you are invaded by the thoughts about eating: sun, flower, seven, path, tee, run, yellow, apple, fish, rain, pen, water, smile, talk, life, sky.
- Think of three different words, any words which just come to your mind at the moment and make a simple story using these 3 words. Repeat untill you fall asleep.

If you cannot fall asleep

- Say slowly whenever you are invaded by the thoughts about eating: sun, flower, seven, path, tee, run, yellow, apple, fish, rain, pen, water, smile, talk, life, sky.

If you cannot asleep

- Think of three different words, any words which just come to your mind at the moment and make a simple story using these 3 words. Repeat untill you fall asleep.

If above does not help

- Stand up and go to the toilet (when possible with as little light as possible)
- Say slowly whenever you are invaded by the thoughts about eating: sun, flower, seven, path,

tee, run, yellow, apple, fish, rain, pen, water, smile, talk, life, sky.
- Think of three different words, any words which just come to your mind at the moment and make a simple story using these 3 words. Repeat untill you fall asleep.

If above does not help
- Say STOP untill you fall asleep

If above does not help
- Go to the kitchen and have a very small snack.
- Back to the bed think of three different words, any words which just come to your mind at the moment and make a simple story using these 3 words. Repeat untill you fall asleep.
- If above does not help think of three different words, any words which just come to your mind at the moment and make a simple story using these 3 words. Repeat untill you fall asleep.
- Say slowly whenever you are invaded by the thoughts about eating: sun, flower, seven, path, tee, run, yellow, apple, fish, rain, pen, water, smile, talk, life, sky. Repeat untill you fall asleep.

***

Day 7

Morning

* Say STOP whenever thoughts about eating come to your mind.

* Say slowly whenever you are invaded by the thoughts about eating: sun, flower, seven, path, tee, run, yellow, apple, fish, rain, pen, water, smile, talk, life, sky.

* If above does not help to stop the thoughts about eating just turn your attention away from the invading thoughts about eating. The best way to turn your attention away from the invading thoughts about eating in your head is by doing one of your favorite occupations. Do not be ashamed of any occupation to turn your attention away from the invading thoughts in your head. ALWAYS be busy with your favorite occupation when unsupportable thoughts come to your head.

* Be careful to keep for yourself these of your believes which are found to be strange by the people.

* CONTROL what you say. Say only things which are not strange for the people. You surely already know which of your believes are found to be strange by the people.

* If you do not know yet which of your believes are found to be strange by the people, OBSERVE how

people react on what you say. If you see that people are ALERTED by your believes, it means your believes are strange. From now on AVOID presenting such believes.

* Think of three different words, any words which just come to your mind at the moment and make a simple story using these 3 words. Repeat 3 times.

* Try to concentrate on an object close to you, any object. What do you feel when looking at the object? What thoughts come to your mind when looking at the object? And why? Maybe there is a reason. Look for the reason but not too long. If you don't find the reason, forget it.

* Small physical excercise (10 min)

* Small breakfast.

* Nice talk (no complaints, no problematic questions) 10 min. When nobody to talk with, phone or internet conversation oral or written.

* Walk 15 min.

* If you have invading thoughts about eating, ask yourself if it is possible to ignore them.

Yes

Great! In such a case continue ignoring them.

No

You have to learn to ignore the invading thoughts about eating.

This Guide will teach you to ignore the invading thoughts about eating.

Remember: even if you cannot stop the invading thoughts, the invading thoughts cannot stop you to live a normal life.

If you believe in things which other people consider strange, try to keep your strange believes for yourself. Everybody has to make the selection of what can be told to other people and what must be private. Believe me, many people have strange believes. Even much stranger than yours. And they are not considered to be sick. Why? Because they keep their strange believes for themselves. That is the secret.

***

Afternoon

* Say slowly whenever you are invaded by the thoughts about eating: sun, flower, seven, path, tee, run, yellow, apple, fish, rain, pen, water, smile, talk, life, sky.

* Think of three different words, any words which just come to your mind at the moment and make a simple story using these 3 words. Repeat 3 times.

* Try to concentrate on an object close to you, any object. What do you feel when looking at the object? What thoughts come to your mind when looking at the object? And why?Maybe there is a reason. Look for the reason but not too long. If you don't find the reason, forget it.

* Dinner and half an hour break (you can sleep).

* Nice talk (no complaints) 15 min. When nobody to talk with, phone or internet conversation oral or written.

* Walk 20 min.

* If you have the invading thoughts about eating, ask yourself if it is possible to ignore them.

Yes

Great! In such a case continue ignoring them.

No

You have to learn to ignore the invading thoughts.

This Guide will teach you to ignore the invading thoughts about eating.

Remember: even if you cannot stop the invading thoughts, the invading thoughts cannot stop you to live a normal life.

If you believe in things which other people consider strange, try to keep your strange believes for yourself. Everybody has to make the selection of what can be told to other people and what must be private. Believe me, many people have strange believes. Even much stranger than yours. And they are not considered to be sick. Why? Because they keep their strange believes for themselves. That is the secret.

***

Evening

- Say slowly whenever you are invaded by the thoughts about eating: sun, flower, seven, path, tee, run, yellow, apple, fish, rain, pen, water, smile, talk, life, sky.

- Think of three different words, any words which just come to your mind at the moment and make a simple story using these 3 words. Repeat 3 times.
  - Try to concentrate on an object close to you, any object. What do you feel when looking at the object? What thoughts come to your mind when

looking at the object? And why? Maybe there is a reason. Look for the reason but not too long. If you don't find the reason, forget it.

- Small supper.
- Nice talk (no complaints) 10 min. When nobody to talk with, phone or internet conversation oral or written.
- Walk 10 min.
- If you have the invading thoughts about eating, ask yourself if it is possible to ignore them.

Yes

Great! In such a case continue ignoring them.

No

You have to learn to ignore the invading thoughts.

This Guide will teach you to ignore the invading thoughts.

Remember: even if you cannot stop the invading thoughts, the invading thoughts cannot stop you to live a normal life.

If you believe in things which other people consider strange, try to keep your strange believes for yourself. Everybody has to make the selection of what can be told to other people and what must be private. Believe

me, many people have strange believes. Even much stranger than yours. And they are not considered to be sick. Why? Because they keep their strange believes for themselves. That is the secret.

***

Night

Before sleep

- Take a shower (warm water) 1 min.
- Small physical excercise 3 min.

In Bed

- Repeat STOP (10 times if you have invading thoughts).
- Say slowly whenever you are invaded by the thoughts about eating: sun, flower, seven, path, tee, run, yellow, apple, fish, rain, pen, water, smile, talk, life, sky.
- Think of three different words, any words which just come to your mind at the moment and make a simple story using these 3 words. Repeat untill you fall asleep.

If you cannot fall asleep

- Say slowly whenever you are invaded by the thoughts about eating: sun, flower, seven, path,

tee, run, yellow, apple, fish, rain, pen, water, smile, talk, life, sky.

If you cannot asleep

- Think of three different words, any words which just come to your mind at the moment and make a simple story using these 3 words. Repeat untill you fall asleep.

If above does not help

- Stand up and go to the toilet (when possible with as little light as possible)
- Say slowly whenever you are invaded by the thoughts about eating: sun, flower, seven, path, tee, run, yellow, apple, fish, rain, pen, water, smile, talk, life, sky.
- Think of three different words, any words which just come to your mind at the moment and make a simple story using these 3 words. Repeat untill you fall asleep.

If above does not help

- Say STOP untill you fall asleep

If above does not help

- Go to the kitchen and have a very small snack.

- Back to the bed think of three different words, any words which just come to your mind at the moment and make a simple story using these 3 words. Repeat untill you fall asleep.
- If above does not help think of three different words, any words which just come to your mind at the moment and make a simple story using these 3 words. Repeat untill you fall asleep.
- Say slowly whenever you are invaded by the thoughts about eating: sun, flower, seven, path, tee, run, yellow, apple, fish, rain, pen, water, smile, talk, life, sky. Repeat untill you fall asleep.

***

Month Two

***

Week Five

Day 1

Morning

* Say STOP whenever thoughts about eating come to your mind.

* Say slowly whenever you are invaded by the thoughts about eating: sun, flower, seven, path, tee, run, yellow, apple, fish, rain, pen, water, smile, talk, life, sky.

* If above does not help to stop the thoughts about eating just turn your attention away from the invading thoughts about eating. The best way to turn your attention away from the invading thoughts about eating in your head is by doing one of your favorite occupations. Do not be ashamed of any occupation to turn your attention away from the invading thoughts in your head. ALWAYS be busy with your favorite occupation when unsupportable thoughts come to your head.

* Be careful to keep for yourself these of your believes which are found to be strange by the people.

* CONTROL what you say. Say only things which are not strange for the people. You surely already know which of your believes are found to be strange by the people.

* If you do not know yet which of your believes are found to be strange by the people, OBSERVE how people react on what you say. If you see that people are ALERTED by your believes, it means your believes are strange. From now on AVOID presenting such believes.

* Think of three different words, any words which just come to your mind at the moment and make a simple story using these 3 words. Repeat 3 times.

* Try to concentrate on an object close to you, any object. What do you feel when looking at the object? What thoughts come to your mind when looking at the object? And why?Maybe there is a reason. Look for the reason but not too long. If you don't find the reason, forget it.

* Small physical excercise (10 min)

* Small breakfast.

* Nice talk (no complaints, no problematic questions) 10 min. When nobody to talk with, phone or internet conversation oral or written.

* Walk 15 min.

* If you have invading thoughts about eating, ask yourself if it is possible to ignore them.

Yes

Great! In such a case continue ignoring them.

No

You have to learn to ignore the invading thoughts about eating.

This Guide will teach you to ignore the invading thoughts about eating.

Remember: even if you cannot stop the invading thoughts, the invading thoughts cannot stop you to live a normal life.

If you believe in things which other people consider strange, try to keep your strange believes for yourself. Everybody has to make the selection of what can be told to other people and what must be private. Believe me, many people have strange believes. Even much stranger than yours. And they are not considered to be sick. Why? Because they keep their strange believes for themselves. That is the secret.

***

Afternoon

* Say slowly whenever you are invaded by the thoughts about eating: sun, flower, seven, path, tee, run, yellow, apple, fish, rain, pen, water, smile, talk, life, sky.

* Think of three different words, any words which just come to your mind at the moment and make a simple story using these 3 words. Repeat 3 times.

* Try to concentrate on an object close to you, any object. What do you feel when looking at the object? What thoughts come to your mind when looking at the

object? And why? Maybe there is a reason. Look for the reason but not too long. If you don't find the reason, forget it.

* Dinner and half an hour break (you can sleep).

* Nice talk (no complaints) 15 min. When nobody to talk with, phone or internet conversation oral or written.

* Walk 20 min.

* If you have the invading thoughts about eating, ask yourself if it is possible to ignore them.

Yes

Great! In such a case continue ignoring them.

No

You have to learn to ignore the invading thoughts.

This Guide will teach you to ignore the invading thoughts about eating.

Remember: even if you cannot stop the invading thoughts, the invading thoughts cannot stop you to live a normal life.

If you believe in things which other people consider strange, try to keep your strange believes for yourself. Everybody has to make the selection of what can be

told to other people and what must be private. Believe me, many people have strange believes. Even much stranger than yours. And they are not considered to be sick. Why? Because they keep their strange believes for themselves. That is the secret.

***

Evening

- Say slowly whenever you are invaded by the thoughts about eating: sun, flower, seven, path, tee, run, yellow, apple, fish, rain, pen, water, smile, talk, life, sky.

- Think of three different words, any words which just come to your mind at the moment and make a simple story using these 3 words. Repeat 3 times.
  - Try to concentrate on an object close to you, any object. What do you feel when looking at the object? What thoughts come to your mind when looking at the object? And why? Maybe there is a reason. Look for the reason but not too long. If you don't find the reason, forget it.
  - Small supper.
  - Nice talk (no complaints) 10 min. When nobody to talk with, phone or internet conversation oral or written.

- Walk 10 min.
- If you have the invading thoughts about eating, ask yourself if it is possible to ignore them.

Yes

Great! In such a case continue ignoring them.

No

You have to learn to ignore the invading thoughts.

This Guide will teach you to ignore the invading thoughts.

Remember: even if you cannot stop the invading thoughts, the invading thoughts cannot stop you to live a normal life.

If you believe in things which other people consider strange, try to keep your strange believes for yourself. Everybody has to make the selection of what can be told to other people and what must be private. Believe me, many people have strange believes. Even much stranger than yours. And they are not considered to be sick. Why? Because they keep their strange believes for themselves. That is the secret.

***

Night

Before sleep
- Take a shower (warm water) 1 min.
- Small physical excercise 3 min.

In Bed
- Repeat STOP (10 times if you have invading thoughts).
- Say slowly whenever you are invaded by the thoughts about eating: sun, flower, seven, path, tee, run, yellow, apple, fish, rain, pen, water, smile, talk, life, sky.
- Think of three different words, any words which just come to your mind at the moment and make a simple story using these 3 words. Repeat untill you fall asleep.

If you cannot fall asleep
- Say slowly whenever you are invaded by the thoughts about eating: sun, flower, seven, path, tee, run, yellow, apple, fish, rain, pen, water, smile, talk, life, sky.

If you cannot asleep
- Think of three different words, any words which just come to your mind at the moment and make a simple story using these 3 words. Repeat untill you fall asleep.

If above does not help

- Stand up and go to the toilet (when possible with as little light as possible)
- Say slowly whenever you are invaded by the thoughts about eating: sun, flower, seven, path, tee, run, yellow, apple, fish, rain, pen, water, smile, talk, life, sky.
- Think of three different words, any words which just come to your mind at the moment and make a simple story using these 3 words. Repeat untill you fall asleep.

If above does not help

- Say STOP untill you fall asleep

If above does not help

- Go to the kitchen and have a very small snack.
- Back to the bed think of three different words, any words which just come to your mind at the moment and make a simple story using these 3 words. Repeat untill you fall asleep.
- If above does not help think of three different words, any words which just come to your mind at the moment and make a simple story using these 3 words. Repeat untill you fall asleep.

- Say slowly whenever you are invaded by the thoughts about eating: sun, flower, seven, path, tee, run, yellow, apple, fish, rain, pen, water, smile, talk, life, sky. Repeat untill you fall asleep.

***

Day 2

Morning

* Say STOP whenever thoughts about eating come to your mind.

* Say slowly whenever you are invaded by the thoughts about eating: sun, flower, seven, path, tee, run, yellow, apple, fish, rain, pen, water, smile, talk, life, sky.

* If above does not help to stop the thoughts about eating just turn your attention away from the invading thoughts about eating. The best way to turn your attention away from the invading thoughts about eating in your head is by doing one of your favorite occupations. Do not be ashamed of any occupation to turn your attention away from the invading thoughts in your head. ALWAYS be busy with your favorite occupation when unsupportable thoughts come to your head.

* Be careful to keep for yourself these of your believes which are found to be strange by the people.

* CONTROL what you say. Say only things which are not strange for the people. You surely already know which of your believes are found to be strange by the people.

* If you do not know yet which of your believes are found to be strange by the people, OBSERVE how people react on what you say. If you see that people are ALERTED by your believes, it means your believes are strange. From now on AVOID presenting such believes.

* Think of three different words, any words which just come to your mind at the moment and make a simple story using these 3 words. Repeat 3 times.

* Try to concentrate on an object close to you, any object. What do you feel when looking at the object? What thoughts come to your mind when looking at the object? And why?Maybe there is a reason. Look for the reason but not too long. If you don't find the reason, forget it.

* Small physical excercise (10 min)

* Small breakfast.

* Nice talk (no complaints, no problematic questions) 10 min. When nobody to talk with, phone or internet conversation oral or written.

* Walk 15 min.

* If you have invading thoughts about eating, ask yourself if it is possible to ignore them.

Yes

Great! In such a case continue ignoring them.

No

You have to learn to ignore the invading thoughts about eating.

This Guide will teach you to ignore the invading thoughts about eating.

Remember: even if you cannot stop the invading thoughts, the invading thoughts cannot stop you to live a normal life.

If you believe in things which other people consider strange, try to keep your strange believes for yourself. Everybody has to make the selection of what can be told to other people and what must be private. Believe me, many people have strange believes. Even much stranger than yours. And they are not considered to be

sick. Why? Because they keep their strange believes for themselves. That is the secret.

***

Afternoon

* Say slowly whenever you are invaded by the thoughts about eating: sun, flower, seven, path, tee, run, yellow, apple, fish, rain, pen, water, smile, talk, life, sky.

* Think of three different words, any words which just come to your mind at the moment and make a simple story using these 3 words. Repeat 3 times.

* Try to concentrate on an object close to you, any object. What do you feel when looking at the object? What thoughts come to your mind when looking at the object? And why?Maybe there is a reason. Look for the reason but not too long. If you don't find the reason, forget it.

* Dinner and half an hour break (you can sleep).

* Nice talk (no complaints) 15 min. When nobody to talk with, phone or internet conversation oral or written.

* Walk 20 min.

* If you have the invading thoughts about eating, ask yourself if it is possible to ignore them.

Yes

Great! In such a case continue ignoring them.

No

You have to learn to ignore the invading thoughts.

This Guide will teach you to ignore the invading thoughts about eating.

Remember: even if you cannot stop the invading thoughts, the invading thoughts cannot stop you to live a normal life.

If you believe in things which other people consider strange, try to keep your strange believes for yourself. Everybody has to make the selection of what can be told to other people and what must be private. Believe me, many people have strange believes. Even much stranger than yours. And they are not considered to be sick. Why? Because they keep their strange believes for themselves. That is the secret.

***

Evening

- Say slowly whenever you are invaded by the thoughts about eating: sun, flower, seven, path, tee, run, yellow, apple, fish, rain, pen, water, smile, talk, life, sky.

- Think of three different words, any words which just come to your mind at the moment and make a simple story using these 3 words. Repeat 3 times.
  - Try to concentrate on an object close to you, any object. What do you feel when looking at the object? What thoughts come to your mind when looking at the object? And why? Maybe there is a reason. Look for the reason but not too long. If you don't find the reason, forget it.
  - Small supper.
  - Nice talk (no complaints) 10 min. When nobody to talk with, phone or internet conversation oral or written.
  - Walk 10 min.
  - If you have the invading thoughts about eating, ask yourself if it is possible to ignore them.

Yes

Great! In such a case continue ignoring them.

No

You have to learn to ignore the invading thoughts.

This Guide will teach you to ignore the invading thoughts.

Remember: even if you cannot stop the invading thoughts, the invading thoughts cannot stop you to live a normal life.

If you believe in things which other people consider strange, try to keep your strange believes for yourself. Everybody has to make the selection of what can be told to other people and what must be private. Believe me, many people have strange believes. Even much stranger than yours. And they are not considered to be sick. Why? Because they keep their strange believes for themselves. That is the secret.

***

Night

Before sleep

- Take a shower (warm water) 1 min.
- Small physical excercise 3 min.

In Bed

- Repeat STOP (10 times if you have invading thoughts).

- Say slowly whenever you are invaded by the thoughts about eating: sun, flower, seven, path, tee, run, yellow, apple, fish, rain, pen, water, smile, talk, life, sky.
- Think of three different words, any words which just come to your mind at the moment and make a simple story using these 3 words. Repeat untill you fall asleep.

If you cannot fall asleep

- Say slowly whenever you are invaded by the thoughts about eating: sun, flower, seven, path, tee, run, yellow, apple, fish, rain, pen, water, smile, talk, life, sky.

If you cannot asleep

- Think of three different words, any words which just come to your mind at the moment and make a simple story using these 3 words. Repeat untill you fall asleep.

If above does not help

- Stand up and go to the toilet (when possible with as little light as possible)
- Say slowly whenever you are invaded by the thoughts about eating: sun, flower, seven, path,

tee, run, yellow, apple, fish, rain, pen, water, smile, talk, life, sky.
- Think of three different words, any words which just come to your mind at the moment and make a simple story using these 3 words. Repeat untill you fall asleep.

If above does not help

- Say STOP untill you fall asleep

If above does not help

- Go to the kitchen and have a very small snack.
- Back to the bed think of three different words, any words which just come to your mind at the moment and make a simple story using these 3 words. Repeat untill you fall asleep.
- If above does not help think of three different words, any words which just come to your mind at the moment and make a simple story using these 3 words. Repeat untill you fall asleep.
- Say slowly whenever you are invaded by the thoughts about eating: sun, flower, seven, path, tee, run, yellow, apple, fish, rain, pen, water, smile, talk, life, sky. Repeat untill you fall asleep.

***

Day 3

Morning

* Say STOP whenever thoughts about eating come to your mind.

* Say slowly whenever you are invaded by the thoughts about eating: sun, flower, seven, path, tee, run, yellow, apple, fish, rain, pen, water, smile, talk, life, sky.

* If above does not help to stop the thoughts about eating just turn your attention away from the invading thoughts about eating. The best way to turn your attention away from the invading thoughts about eating in your head is by doing one of your favorite occupations. Do not be ashamed of any occupation to turn your attention away from the invading thoughts in your head. ALWAYS be busy with your favorite occupation when unsupportable thoughts come to your head.

* Be careful to keep for yourself these of your believes which are found to be strange by the people.

* CONTROL what you say. Say only things which are not strange for the people. You surely already know which of your believes are found to be strange by the people.

* If you do not know yet which of your believes are found to be strange by the people, OBSERVE how

people react on what you say. If you see that people are ALERTED by your believes, it means your believes are strange. From now on AVOID presenting such believes.

* Think of three different words, any words which just come to your mind at the moment and make a simple story using these 3 words. Repeat 3 times.

* Try to concentrate on an object close to you, any object. What do you feel when looking at the object? What thoughts come to your mind when looking at the object? And why? Maybe there is a reason. Look for the reason but not too long. If you don't find the reason, forget it.

* Small physical excercise (10 min)

* Small breakfast.

* Nice talk (no complaints, no problematic questions) 10 min. When nobody to talk with, phone or internet conversation oral or written.

* Walk 15 min.

* If you have invading thoughts about eating, ask yourself if it is possible to ignore them.

Yes

Great! In such a case continue ignoring them.

No

You have to learn to ignore the invading thoughts about eating.

This Guide will teach you to ignore the invading thoughts about eating.

Remember: even if you cannot stop the invading thoughts, the invading thoughts cannot stop you to live a normal life.

If you believe in things which other people consider strange, try to keep your strange believes for yourself. Everybody has to make the selection of what can be told to other people and what must be private. Believe me, many people have strange believes. Even much stranger than yours. And they are not considered to be sick. Why? Because they keep their strange believes for themselves. That is the secret.

***

Afternoon

* Say slowly whenever you are invaded by the thoughts about eating: sun, flower, seven, path, tee, run, yellow, apple, fish, rain, pen, water, smile, talk, life, sky.

* Think of three different words, any words which just come to your mind at the moment and make a simple story using these 3 words. Repeat 3 times.

* Try to concentrate on an object close to you, any object. What do you feel when looking at the object? What thoughts come to your mind when looking at the object? And why? Maybe there is a reason. Look for the reason but not too long. If you don't find the reason, forget it.

* Dinner and half an hour break (you can sleep).

* Nice talk (no complaints) 15 min. When nobody to talk with, phone or internet conversation oral or written.

* Walk 20 min.

* If you have the invading thoughts about eating, ask yourself if it is possible to ignore them.

Yes

Great! In such a case continue ignoring them.

No

You have to learn to ignore the invading thoughts.

This Guide will teach you to ignore the invading thoughts about eating.

Remember: even if you cannot stop the invading thoughts, the invading thoughts cannot stop you to live a normal life.

If you believe in things which other people consider strange, try to keep your strange believes for yourself. Everybody has to make the selection of what can be told to other people and what must be private. Believe me, many people have strange believes. Even much stranger than yours. And they are not considered to be sick. Why? Because they keep their strange believes for themselves. That is the secret.

***

Evening

- Say slowly whenever you are invaded by the thoughts about eating: sun, flower, seven, path, tee, run, yellow, apple, fish, rain, pen, water, smile, talk, life, sky.

- Think of three different words, any words which just come to your mind at the moment and make a simple story using these 3 words. Repeat 3 times.
  - Try to concentrate on an object close to you, any object. What do you feel when looking at the object? What thoughts come to your mind when

looking at the object? And why? Maybe there is a reason. Look for the reason but not too long. If you don't find the reason, forget it.

- Small supper.
- Nice talk (no complaints) 10 min. When nobody to talk with, phone or internet conversation oral or written.
- Walk 10 min.
- If you have the invading thoughts about eating, ask yourself if it is possible to ignore them.

Yes

Great! In such a case continue ignoring them.

No

You have to learn to ignore the invading thoughts.

This Guide will teach you to ignore the invading thoughts.

Remember: even if you cannot stop the invading thoughts, the invading thoughts cannot stop you to live a normal life.

If you believe in things which other people consider strange, try to keep your strange believes for yourself. Everybody has to make the selection of what can be told to other people and what must be private. Believe

me, many people have strange believes. Even much stranger than yours. And they are not considered to be sick. Why? Because they keep their strange believes for themselves. That is the secret.

***

Night

Before sleep

- Take a shower (warm water) 1 min.
- Small physical excercise 3 min.

In Bed

- Repeat STOP (10 times if you have invading thoughts).
- Say slowly whenever you are invaded by the thoughts about eating: sun, flower, seven, path, tee, run, yellow, apple, fish, rain, pen, water, smile, talk, life, sky.
- Think of three different words, any words which just come to your mind at the moment and make a simple story using these 3 words. Repeat untill you fall asleep.

If you cannot fall asleep

- Say slowly whenever you are invaded by the thoughts about eating: sun, flower, seven, path,

tee, run, yellow, apple, fish, rain, pen, water, smile, talk, life, sky.

If you cannot asleep

- Think of three different words, any words which just come to your mind at the moment and make a simple story using these 3 words. Repeat untill you fall asleep.

If above does not help

- Stand up and go to the toilet (when possible with as little light as possible)
- Say slowly whenever you are invaded by the thoughts about eating: sun, flower, seven, path, tee, run, yellow, apple, fish, rain, pen, water, smile, talk, life, sky.
- Think of three different words, any words which just come to your mind at the moment and make a simple story using these 3 words. Repeat untill you fall asleep.

If above does not help

- Say STOP untill you fall asleep

If above does not help

- Go to the kitchen and have a very small snack.

- Back to the bed think of three different words, any words which just come to your mind at the moment and make a simple story using these 3 words. Repeat untill you fall asleep.
- If above does not help think of three different words, any words which just come to your mind at the moment and make a simple story using these 3 words. Repeat untill you fall asleep.
- Say slowly whenever you are invaded by the thoughts about eating: sun, flower, seven, path, tee, run, yellow, apple, fish, rain, pen, water, smile, talk, life, sky. Repeat untill you fall asleep.

***

Day 4

Morning

* Say STOP whenever thoughts about eating come to your mind.

* Say slowly whenever you are invaded by the thoughts about eating: sun, flower, seven, path, tee, run, yellow, apple, fish, rain, pen, water, smile, talk, life, sky.

* If above does not help to stop the thoughts about eating just turn your attention away from the invading thoughts about eating. The best way to turn your

attention away from the invading thoughts about eating in your head is by doing one of your favorite occupations. Do not be ashamed of any occupation to turn your attention away from the invading thoughts in your head. ALWAYS be busy with your favorite occupation when unsupportable thoughts come to your head.

* Be careful to keep for yourself these of your believes which are found to be strange by the people.

* CONTROL what you say. Say only things which are not strange for the people. You surely already know which of your believes are found to be strange by the people.

* If you do not know yet which of your believes are found to be strange by the people, OBSERVE how people react on what you say. If you see that people are ALERTED by your believes, it means your believes are strange. From now on AVOID presenting such believes.

* Think of three different words, any words which just come to your mind at the moment and make a simple story using these 3 words. Repeat 3 times.

* Try to concentrate on an object close to you, any object. What do you feel when looking at the object? What thoughts come to your mind when looking at the object? And why? Maybe there is a reason. Look for the

reason but not too long. If you don't find the reason, forget it.

* Small physical excercise (10 min)

* Small breakfast.

* Nice talk (no complaints, no problematic questions) 10 min. When nobody to talk with, phone or internet conversation oral or written.

* Walk 15 min.

* If you have invading thoughts about eating, ask yourself if it is possible to ignore them.

Yes

Great! In such a case continue ignoring them.

No

You have to learn to ignore the invading thoughts about eating.

This Guide will teach you to ignore the invading thoughts about eating.

Remember: even if you cannot stop the invading thoughts, the invading thoughts cannot stop you to live a normal life.

If you believe in things which other people consider strange, try to keep your strange believes for yourself. Everybody has to make the selection of what can be told to other people and what must be private. Believe me, many people have strange believes. Even much stranger than yours. And they are not considered to be sick. Why? Because they keep their strange believes for themselves. That is the secret.

***

Afternoon

* Say slowly whenever you are invaded by the thoughts about eating: sun, flower, seven, path, tee, run, yellow, apple, fish, rain, pen, water, smile, talk, life, sky.

* Think of three different words, any words which just come to your mind at the moment and make a simple story using these 3 words. Repeat 3 times.

* Try to concentrate on an object close to you, any object. What do you feel when looking at the object? What thoughts come to your mind when looking at the object? And why? Maybe there is a reason. Look for the reason but not too long. If you don't find the reason, forget it.

* Dinner and half an hour break (you can sleep).

* Nice talk (no complaints) 15 min. When nobody to talk with, phone or internet conversation oral or written.

* Walk 20 min.

* If you have the invading thoughts about eating, ask yourself if it is possible to ignore them.

Yes

Great! In such a case continue ignoring them.

No

You have to learn to ignore the invading thoughts.

This Guide will teach you to ignore the invading thoughts about eating.

Remember: even if you cannot stop the invading thoughts, the invading thoughts cannot stop you to live a normal life.

If you believe in things which other people consider strange, try to keep your strange believes for yourself. Everybody has to make the selection of what can be told to other people and what must be private. Believe me, many people have strange believes. Even much stranger than yours. And they are not considered to be

sick. Why? Because they keep their strange believes for themselves. That is the secret.

***

Evening

- Say slowly whenever you are invaded by the thoughts about eating: sun, flower, seven, path, tee, run, yellow, apple, fish, rain, pen, water, smile, talk, life, sky.

- Think of three different words, any words which just come to your mind at the moment and make a simple story using these 3 words. Repeat 3 times.
  - Try to concentrate on an object close to you, any object. What do you feel when looking at the object? What thoughts come to your mind when looking at the object? And why? Maybe there is a reason. Look for the reason but not too long. If you don't find the reason, forget it.
  - Small supper.
  - Nice talk (no complaints) 10 min. When nobody to talk with, phone or internet conversation oral or written.
  - Walk 10 min.
  - If you have the invading thoughts about eating, ask yourself if it is possible to ignore them.

Yes

Great! In such a case continue ignoring them.

No

You have to learn to ignore the invading thoughts.

This Guide will teach you to ignore the invading thoughts.

Remember: even if you cannot stop the invading thoughts, the invading thoughts cannot stop you to live a normal life.

If you believe in things which other people consider strange, try to keep your strange believes for yourself. Everybody has to make the selection of what can be told to other people and what must be private. Believe me, many people have strange believes. Even much stranger than yours. And they are not considered to be sick. Why? Because they keep their strange believes for themselves. That is the secret.

***

Night

Before sleep

- Take a shower (warm water) 1 min.
- Small physical excercise 3 min.

In Bed

- Repeat STOP (10 times if you have invading thoughts).
- Say slowly whenever you are invaded by the thoughts about eating: sun, flower, seven, path, tee, run, yellow, apple, fish, rain, pen, water, smile, talk, life, sky.
- Think of three different words, any words which just come to your mind at the moment and make a simple story using these 3 words. Repeat untill you fall asleep.

If you cannot fall asleep

- Say slowly whenever you are invaded by the thoughts about eating: sun, flower, seven, path, tee, run, yellow, apple, fish, rain, pen, water, smile, talk, life, sky.

If you cannot asleep

- Think of three different words, any words which just come to your mind at the moment and make a simple story using these 3 words. Repeat untill you fall asleep.

If above does not help

- Stand up and go to the toilet (when possible with as little light as possible)

- Say slowly whenever you are invaded by the thoughts about eating: sun, flower, seven, path, tee, run, yellow, apple, fish, rain, pen, water, smile, talk, life, sky.
- Think of three different words, any words which just come to your mind at the moment and make a simple story using these 3 words. Repeat untill you fall asleep.

If above does not help

- Say STOP untill you fall asleep

If above does not help

- Go to the kitchen and have a very small snack.
- Back to the bed think of three different words, any words which just come to your mind at the moment and make a simple story using these 3 words. Repeat untill you fall asleep.
- If above does not help think of three different words, any words which just come to your mind at the moment and make a simple story using these 3 words. Repeat untill you fall asleep.
- Say slowly whenever you are invaded by the thoughts about eating: sun, flower, seven, path, tee, run, yellow, apple, fish, rain, pen, water, smile, talk, life, sky. Repeat untill you fall asleep.

***

Day 5

Morning

* Say STOP whenever thoughts about eating come to your mind.

* Say slowly whenever you are invaded by the thoughts about eating: sun, flower, seven, path, tee, run, yellow, apple, fish, rain, pen, water, smile, talk, life, sky.

* If above does not help to stop the thoughts about eating just turn your attention away from the invading thoughts about eating. The best way to turn your attention away from the invading thoughts about eating in your head is by doing one of your favorite occupations. Do not be ashamed of any occupation to turn your attention away from the invading thoughts in your head. ALWAYS be busy with your favorite occupation when unsupportable thoughts come to your head.

* Be careful to keep for yourself these of your believes which are found to be strange by the people.

* CONTROL what you say. Say only things which are not strange for the people. You surely already know which of your believes are found to be strange by the people.

* If you do not know yet which of your believes are found to be strange by the people, OBSERVE how people react on what you say. If you see that people are ALERTED by your believes, it means your believes are strange. From now on AVOID presenting such believes.

* Think of three different words, any words which just come to your mind at the moment and make a simple story using these 3 words. Repeat 3 times.

* Try to concentrate on an object close to you, any object. What do you feel when looking at the object? What thoughts come to your mind when looking at the object? And why? Maybe there is a reason. Look for the reason but not too long. If you don't find the reason, forget it.

* Small physical excercise (10 min)

* Small breakfast.

* Nice talk (no complaints, no problematic questions) 10 min. When nobody to talk with, phone or internet conversation oral or written.

* Walk 15 min.

* If you have invading thoughts about eating, ask yourself if it is possible to ignore them.

Yes

Great! In such a case continue ignoring them.

No

You have to learn to ignore the invading thoughts about eating.

This Guide will teach you to ignore the invading thoughts about eating.

Remember: even if you cannot stop the invading thoughts, the invading thoughts cannot stop you to live a normal life.

If you believe in things which other people consider strange, try to keep your strange believes for yourself. Everybody has to make the selection of what can be told to other people and what must be private. Believe me, many people have strange believes. Even much stranger than yours. And they are not considered to be sick. Why? Because they keep their strange believes for themselves. That is the secret.

***

Afternoon

* Say slowly whenever you are invaded by the thoughts about eating: sun, flower, seven, path, tee, run, yellow, apple, fish, rain, pen, water, smile, talk, life, sky.

* Think of three different words, any words which just come to your mind at the moment and make a simple story using these 3 words. Repeat 3 times.

* Try to concentrate on an object close to you, any object. What do you feel when looking at the object? What thoughts come to your mind when looking at the object? And why? Maybe there is a reason. Look for the reason but not too long. If you don't find the reason, forget it.

* Dinner and half an hour break (you can sleep).

* Nice talk (no complaints) 15 min. When nobody to talk with, phone or internet conversation oral or written.

* Walk 20 min.

* If you have the invading thoughts about eating, ask yourself if it is possible to ignore them.

Yes

Great! In such a case continue ignoring them.

No

You have to learn to ignore the invading thoughts.

This Guide will teach you to ignore the invading thoughts about eating.

Remember: even if you cannot stop the invading thoughts, the invading thoughts cannot stop you to live a normal life.

If you believe in things which other people consider strange, try to keep your strange believes for yourself. Everybody has to make the selection of what can be told to other people and what must be private. Believe me, many people have strange believes. Even much stranger than yours. And they are not considered to be sick. Why? Because they keep their strange believes for themselves. That is the secret.

***

Evening

- Say slowly whenever you are invaded by the thoughts about eating: sun, flower, seven, path, tee, run, yellow, apple, fish, rain, pen, water, smile, talk, life, sky.

- Think of three different words, any words which just come to your mind at the moment and make a simple story using these 3 words. Repeat 3 times.

- Try to concentrate on an object close to you, any object. What do you feel when looking at the object? What thoughts come to your mind when looking at the object? And why? Maybe there is a reason. Look for the reason but not too long. If you don't find the reason, forget it.
- Small supper.
- Nice talk (no complaints) 10 min. When nobody to talk with, phone or internet conversation oral or written.
- Walk 10 min.
- If you have the invading thoughts about eating, ask yourself if it is possible to ignore them.

Yes

Great! In such a case continue ignoring them.

No

You have to learn to ignore the invading thoughts.

This Guide will teach you to ignore the invading thoughts.

Remember: even if you cannot stop the invading thoughts, the invading thoughts cannot stop you to live a normal life.

If you believe in things which other people consider strange, try to keep your strange believes for yourself. Everybody has to make the selection of what can be told to other people and what must be private. Believe me, many people have strange believes. Even much stranger than yours. And they are not considered to be sick. Why? Because they keep their strange believes for themselves. That is the secret.

***

Night

Before sleep

- Take a shower (warm water) 1 min.
- Small physical excercise 3 min.

In Bed

- Repeat STOP (10 times if you have invading thoughts).
- Say slowly whenever you are invaded by the thoughts about eating: sun, flower, seven, path, tee, run, yellow, apple, fish, rain, pen, water, smile, talk, life, sky.
- Think of three different words, any words which just come to your mind at the moment and make a simple story using these 3 words. Repeat untill you fall asleep.

If you cannot fall asleep

- Say slowly whenever you are invaded by the thoughts about eating: sun, flower, seven, path, tee, run, yellow, apple, fish, rain, pen, water, smile, talk, life, sky.

If you cannot asleep

- Think of three different words, any words which just come to your mind at the moment and make a simple story using these 3 words. Repeat untill you fall asleep.

If above does not help

- Stand up and go to the toilet (when possible with as little light as possible)
- Say slowly whenever you are invaded by the thoughts about eating: sun, flower, seven, path, tee, run, yellow, apple, fish, rain, pen, water, smile, talk, life, sky.
- Think of three different words, any words which just come to your mind at the moment and make a simple story using these 3 words. Repeat untill you fall asleep.

If above does not help

- Say STOP untill you fall asleep

If above does not help

- Go to the kitchen and have a very small snack.
- Back to the bed think of three different words, any words which just come to your mind at the moment and make a simple story using these 3 words. Repeat untill you fall asleep.
- If above does not help think of three different words, any words which just come to your mind at the moment and make a simple story using these 3 words. Repeat untill you fall asleep.
- Say slowly whenever you are invaded by the thoughts about eating: sun, flower, seven, path, tee, run, yellow, apple, fish, rain, pen, water, smile, talk, life, sky. Repeat untill you fall asleep.

***

Day 6

Morning

* Say STOP whenever thoughts about eating come to your mind.

* Say slowly whenever you are invaded by the thoughts about eating: sun, flower, seven, path, tee, run, yellow, apple, fish, rain, pen, water, smile, talk, life, sky.

* If above does not help to stop the thoughts about eating just turn your attention away from the invading thoughts about eating. The best way to turn your attention away from the invading thoughts about eating in your head is by doing one of your favorite occupations. Do not be ashamed of any occupation to turn your attention away from the invading thoughts in your head. ALWAYS be busy with your favorite occupation when unsupportable thoughts come to your head.

* Be careful to keep for yourself these of your believes which are found to be strange by the people.

* CONTROL what you say. Say only things which are not strange for the people. You surely already know which of your believes are found to be strange by the people.

* If you do not know yet which of your believes are found to be strange by the people, OBSERVE how people react on what you say. If you see that people are ALERTED by your believes, it means your believes are strange. From now on AVOID presenting such believes.

* Think of three different words, any words which just come to your mind at the moment and make a simple story using these 3 words. Repeat 3 times.

* Try to concentrate on an object close to you, any object. What do you feel when looking at the object? What thoughts come to your mind when looking at the object? And why? Maybe there is a reason. Look for the reason but not too long. If you don't find the reason, forget it.

* Small physical excercise (10 min)

* Small breakfast.

* Nice talk (no complaints, no problematic questions) 10 min. When nobody to talk with, phone or internet conversation oral or written.

* Walk 15 min.

* If you have invading thoughts about eating, ask yourself if it is possible to ignore them.

Yes

Great! In such a case continue ignoring them.

No

You have to learn to ignore the invading thoughts about eating.

This Guide will teach you to ignore the invading thoughts about eating.

Remember: even if you cannot stop the invading thoughts, the invading thoughts cannot stop you to live a normal life.

If you believe in things which other people consider strange, try to keep your strange believes for yourself. Everybody has to make the selection of what can be told to other people and what must be private. Believe me, many people have strange believes. Even much stranger than yours. And they are not considered to be sick. Why? Because they keep their strange believes for themselves. That is the secret.

***

Afternoon

* Say slowly whenever you are invaded by the thoughts about eating: sun, flower, seven, path, tee, run, yellow, apple, fish, rain, pen, water, smile, talk, life, sky.

* Think of three different words, any words which just come to your mind at the moment and make a simple story using these 3 words. Repeat 3 times.

* Try to concentrate on an object close to you, any object. What do you feel when looking at the object? What thoughts come to your mind when looking at the

object? And why? Maybe there is a reason. Look for the reason but not too long. If you don't find the reason, forget it.

* Dinner and half an hour break (you can sleep).

* Nice talk (no complaints) 15 min. When nobody to talk with, phone or internet conversation oral or written.

* Walk 20 min.

* If you have the invading thoughts about eating, ask yourself if it is possible to ignore them.

Yes

Great! In such a case continue ignoring them.

No

You have to learn to ignore the invading thoughts.

This Guide will teach you to ignore the invading thoughts about eating.

Remember: even if you cannot stop the invading thoughts, the invading thoughts cannot stop you to live a normal life.

If you believe in things which other people consider strange, try to keep your strange believes for yourself. Everybody has to make the selection of what can be

told to other people and what must be private. Believe me, many people have strange believes. Even much stranger than yours. And they are not considered to be sick. Why? Because they keep their strange believes for themselves. That is the secret.

***

Evening

- Say slowly whenever you are invaded by the thoughts about eating: sun, flower, seven, path, tee, run, yellow, apple, fish, rain, pen, water, smile, talk, life, sky.

- Think of three different words, any words which just come to your mind at the moment and make a simple story using these 3 words. Repeat 3 times.
  - Try to concentrate on an object close to you, any object. What do you feel when looking at the object? What thoughts come to your mind when looking at the object? And why? Maybe there is a reason. Look for the reason but not too long. If you don't find the reason, forget it.
  - Small supper.
  - Nice talk (no complaints) 10 min. When nobody to talk with, phone or internet conversation oral or written.

- Walk 10 min.
- If you have the invading thoughts about eating, ask yourself if it is possible to ignore them.

Yes

Great! In such a case continue ignoring them.

No

You have to learn to ignore the invading thoughts.

This Guide will teach you to ignore the invading thoughts.

Remember: even if you cannot stop the invading thoughts, the invading thoughts cannot stop you to live a normal life.

If you believe in things which other people consider strange, try to keep your strange believes for yourself. Everybody has to make the selection of what can be told to other people and what must be private. Believe me, many people have strange believes. Even much stranger than yours. And they are not considered to be sick. Why? Because they keep their strange believes for themselves. That is the secret.

***

Night

Before sleep

- Take a shower (warm water) 1 min.
- Small physical excercise 3 min.

In Bed

- Repeat STOP (10 times if you have invading thoughts).
- Say slowly whenever you are invaded by the thoughts about eating: sun, flower, seven, path, tee, run, yellow, apple, fish, rain, pen, water, smile, talk, life, sky.
- Think of three different words, any words which just come to your mind at the moment and make a simple story using these 3 words. Repeat untill you fall asleep.

If you cannot fall asleep

- Say slowly whenever you are invaded by the thoughts about eating: sun, flower, seven, path, tee, run, yellow, apple, fish, rain, pen, water, smile, talk, life, sky.

If you cannot asleep

- Think of three different words, any words which just come to your mind at the moment and make a simple story using these 3 words. Repeat untill you fall asleep.

If above does not help

- Stand up and go to the toilet (when possible with as little light as possible)
- Say slowly whenever you are invaded by the thoughts about eating: sun, flower, seven, path, tee, run, yellow, apple, fish, rain, pen, water, smile, talk, life, sky.
- Think of three different words, any words which just come to your mind at the moment and make a simple story using these 3 words. Repeat untill you fall asleep.

If above does not help

- Say STOP untill you fall asleep

If above does not help

- Go to the kitchen and have a very small snack.
- Back to the bed think of three different words, any words which just come to your mind at the moment and make a simple story using these 3 words. Repeat untill you fall asleep.
- If above does not help think of three different words, any words which just come to your mind at the moment and make a simple story using these 3 words. Repeat untill you fall asleep.

- Say slowly whenever you are invaded by the thoughts about eating: sun, flower, seven, path, tee, run, yellow, apple, fish, rain, pen, water, smile, talk, life, sky. Repeat untill you fall asleep.

***

Day 7

Morning

* Say STOP whenever thoughts about eating come to your mind.

* Say slowly whenever you are invaded by the thoughts about eating: sun, flower, seven, path, tee, run, yellow, apple, fish, rain, pen, water, smile, talk, life, sky.

* If above does not help to stop the thoughts about eating just turn your attention away from the invading thoughts about eating. The best way to turn your attention away from the invading thoughts about eating in your head is by doing one of your favorite occupations. Do not be ashamed of any occupation to turn your attention away from the invading thoughts in your head. ALWAYS be busy with your favorite occupation when unsupportable thoughts come to your head.

* Be careful to keep for yourself these of your believes which are found to be strange by the people.

* CONTROL what you say. Say only things which are not strange for the people. You surely already know which of your believes are found to be strange by the people.

* If you do not know yet which of your believes are found to be strange by the people, OBSERVE how people react on what you say. If you see that people are ALERTED by your believes, it means your believes are strange. From now on AVOID presenting such believes.

* Think of three different words, any words which just come to your mind at the moment and make a simple story using these 3 words. Repeat 3 times.

* Try to concentrate on an object close to you, any object. What do you feel when looking at the object? What thoughts come to your mind when looking at the object? And why?Maybe there is a reason. Look for the reason but not too long. If you don't find the reason, forget it.

* Small physical excercise (10 min)

* Small breakfast.

* Nice talk (no complaints, no problematic questions) 10 min. When nobody to talk with, phone or internet conversation oral or written.

* Walk 15 min.

* If you have invading thoughts about eating, ask yourself if it is possible to ignore them.

Yes

Great! In such a case continue ignoring them.

No

You have to learn to ignore the invading thoughts about eating.

This Guide will teach you to ignore the invading thoughts about eating.

Remember: even if you cannot stop the invading thoughts, the invading thoughts cannot stop you to live a normal life.

If you believe in things which other people consider strange, try to keep your strange believes for yourself. Everybody has to make the selection of what can be told to other people and what must be private. Believe me, many people have strange believes. Even much stranger than yours. And they are not considered to be

sick. Why? Because they keep their strange believes for themselves. That is the secret.

***

Afternoon

* Say slowly whenever you are invaded by the thoughts about eating: sun, flower, seven, path, tee, run, yellow, apple, fish, rain, pen, water, smile, talk, life, sky.

* Think of three different words, any words which just come to your mind at the moment and make a simple story using these 3 words. Repeat 3 times.

* Try to concentrate on an object close to you, any object. What do you feel when looking at the object? What thoughts come to your mind when looking at the object? And why? Maybe there is a reason. Look for the reason but not too long. If you don't find the reason, forget it.

* Dinner and half an hour break (you can sleep).

* Nice talk (no complaints) 15 min. When nobody to talk with, phone or internet conversation oral or written.

* Walk 20 min.

* If you have the invading thoughts about eating, ask yourself if it is possible to ignore them.

Yes

Great! In such a case continue ignoring them.

No

You have to learn to ignore the invading thoughts.

This Guide will teach you to ignore the invading thoughts about eating.

Remember: even if you cannot stop the invading thoughts, the invading thoughts cannot stop you to live a normal life.

If you believe in things which other people consider strange, try to keep your strange believes for yourself. Everybody has to make the selection of what can be told to other people and what must be private. Believe me, many people have strange believes. Even much stranger than yours. And they are not considered to be sick. Why? Because they keep their strange believes for themselves. That is the secret.

***

Evening

- Say slowly whenever you are invaded by the thoughts about eating: sun, flower, seven, path, tee, run, yellow, apple, fish, rain, pen, water, smile, talk, life, sky.

- Think of three different words, any words which just come to your mind at the moment and make a simple story using these 3 words. Repeat 3 times.
  - Try to concentrate on an object close to you, any object. What do you feel when looking at the object? What thoughts come to your mind when looking at the object? And why? Maybe there is a reason. Look for the reason but not too long. If you don't find the reason, forget it.
  - Small supper.
  - Nice talk (no complaints) 10 min. When nobody to talk with, phone or internet conversation oral or written.
  - Walk 10 min.
  - If you have the invading thoughts about eating, ask yourself if it is possible to ignore them.

Yes

Great! In such a case continue ignoring them.

No

You have to learn to ignore the invading thoughts.

This Guide will teach you to ignore the invading thoughts.

Remember: even if you cannot stop the invading thoughts, the invading thoughts cannot stop you to live a normal life.

If you believe in things which other people consider strange, try to keep your strange believes for yourself. Everybody has to make the selection of what can be told to other people and what must be private. Believe me, many people have strange believes. Even much stranger than yours. And they are not considered to be sick. Why? Because they keep their strange believes for themselves. That is the secret.

***

Night

Before sleep

- Take a shower (warm water) 1 min.
- Small physical excercise 3 min.

In Bed

- Repeat STOP (10 times if you have invading thoughts).

- Say slowly whenever you are invaded by the thoughts about eating: sun, flower, seven, path, tee, run, yellow, apple, fish, rain, pen, water, smile, talk, life, sky.
- Think of three different words, any words which just come to your mind at the moment and make a simple story using these 3 words. Repeat untill you fall asleep.

If you cannot fall asleep

- Say slowly whenever you are invaded by the thoughts about eating: sun, flower, seven, path, tee, run, yellow, apple, fish, rain, pen, water, smile, talk, life, sky.

If you cannot asleep

- Think of three different words, any words which just come to your mind at the moment and make a simple story using these 3 words. Repeat untill you fall asleep.

If above does not help

- Stand up and go to the toilet (when possible with as little light as possible)
- Say slowly whenever you are invaded by the thoughts about eating: sun, flower, seven, path,

tee, run, yellow, apple, fish, rain, pen, water, smile, talk, life, sky.
- Think of three different words, any words which just come to your mind at the moment and make a simple story using these 3 words. Repeat untill you fall asleep.

If above does not help
- Say STOP untill you fall asleep

If above does not help
- Go to the kitchen and have a very small snack.
- Back to the bed think of three different words, any words which just come to your mind at the moment and make a simple story using these 3 words. Repeat untill you fall asleep.
- If above does not help think of three different words, any words which just come to your mind at the moment and make a simple story using these 3 words. Repeat untill you fall asleep.
- Say slowly whenever you are invaded by the thoughts about eating: sun, flower, seven, path, tee, run, yellow, apple, fish, rain, pen, water, smile, talk, life, sky. Repeat untill you fall asleep.

***

Week Six

Day 1

Morning

* Say STOP whenever thoughts about eating come to your mind.

* Say slowly whenever you are invaded by the thoughts about eating: sun, flower, seven, path, tee, run, yellow, apple, fish, rain, pen, water, smile, talk, life, sky.

* If above does not help to stop the thoughts about eating just turn your attention away from the invading thoughts about eating. The best way to turn your attention away from the invading thoughts about eating in your head is by doing one of your favorite occupations. Do not be ashamed of any occupation to turn your attention away from the invading thoughts in your head. ALWAYS be busy with your favorite occupation when unsupportable thoughts come to your head.

* Be careful to keep for yourself these of your believes which are found to be strange by the people.

* CONTROL what you say. Say only things which are not strange for the people. You surely already know which of your believes are found to be strange by the people.

* If you do not know yet which of your believes are found to be strange by the people, OBSERVE how people react on what you say. If you see that people are ALERTED by your believes, it means your believes are strange. From now on AVOID presenting such believes.

* Think of three different words, any words which just come to your mind at the moment and make a simple story using these 3 words. Repeat 3 times.

* Try to concentrate on an object close to you, any object. What do you feel when looking at the object? What thoughts come to your mind when looking at the object? And why?Maybe there is a reason. Look for the reason but not too long. If you don't find the reason, forget it.

* Small physical excercise (10 min)

* Small breakfast.

* Nice talk (no complaints, no problematic questions) 10 min. When nobody to talk with, phone or internet conversation oral or written.

* Walk 15 min.

* If you have invading thoughts about eating, ask yourself if it is possible to ignore them.

Yes

Great! In such a case continue ignoring them.

No

You have to learn to ignore the invading thoughts about eating.

This Guide will teach you to ignore the invading thoughts about eating.

Remember: even if you cannot stop the invading thoughts, the invading thoughts cannot stop you to live a normal life.

If you believe in things which other people consider strange, try to keep your strange believes for yourself. Everybody has to make the selection of what can be told to other people and what must be private. Believe me, many people have strange believes. Even much stranger than yours. And they are not considered to be sick. Why? Because they keep their strange believes for themselves. That is the secret.

***

Afternoon

* Say slowly whenever you are invaded by the thoughts about eating: sun, flower, seven, path, tee, run, yellow, apple, fish, rain, pen, water, smile, talk, life, sky.

* Think of three different words, any words which just come to your mind at the moment and make a simple story using these 3 words. Repeat 3 times.

* Try to concentrate on an object close to you, any object. What do you feel when looking at the object? What thoughts come to your mind when looking at the object? And why? Maybe there is a reason. Look for the reason but not too long. If you don't find the reason, forget it.

* Dinner and half an hour break (you can sleep).

* Nice talk (no complaints) 15 min. When nobody to talk with, phone or internet conversation oral or written.

* Walk 20 min.

* If you have the invading thoughts about eating, ask yourself if it is possible to ignore them.

Yes

Great! In such a case continue ignoring them.

No

You have to learn to ignore the invading thoughts.

This Guide will teach you to ignore the invading thoughts about eating.

Remember: even if you cannot stop the invading thoughts, the invading thoughts cannot stop you to live a normal life.

If you believe in things which other people consider strange, try to keep your strange believes for yourself. Everybody has to make the selection of what can be told to other people and what must be private. Believe me, many people have strange believes. Even much stranger than yours. And they are not considered to be sick. Why? Because they keep their strange believes for themselves. That is the secret.

***

Evening

- Say slowly whenever you are invaded by the thoughts about eating: sun, flower, seven, path, tee, run, yellow, apple, fish, rain, pen, water, smile, talk, life, sky.

- Think of three different words, any words which just come to your mind at the moment and make a simple story using these 3 words. Repeat 3 times.

- Try to concentrate on an object close to you, any object. What do you feel when looking at the object? What thoughts come to your mind when looking at the object? And why? Maybe there is a reason. Look for the reason but not too long. If you don't find the reason, forget it.
- Small supper.
- Nice talk (no complaints) 10 min. When nobody to talk with, phone or internet conversation oral or written.
- Walk 10 min.
- If you have the invading thoughts about eating, ask yourself if it is possible to ignore them.

Yes

Great! In such a case continue ignoring them.

No

You have to learn to ignore the invading thoughts.

This Guide will teach you to ignore the invading thoughts.

Remember: even if you cannot stop the invading thoughts, the invading thoughts cannot stop you to live a normal life.

If you believe in things which other people consider strange, try to keep your strange believes for yourself. Everybody has to make the selection of what can be told to other people and what must be private. Believe me, many people have strange believes. Even much stranger than yours. And they are not considered to be sick. Why? Because they keep their strange believes for themselves. That is the secret.

***

Night

Before sleep

- Take a shower (warm water) 1 min.
- Small physical excercise 3 min.

In Bed

- Repeat STOP (10 times if you have invading thoughts).
- Say slowly whenever you are invaded by the thoughts about eating: sun, flower, seven, path, tee, run, yellow, apple, fish, rain, pen, water, smile, talk, life, sky.
- Think of three different words, any words which just come to your mind at the moment and make a simple story using these 3 words. Repeat untill you fall asleep.

If you cannot fall asleep

- Say slowly whenever you are invaded by the thoughts about eating: sun, flower, seven, path, tee, run, yellow, apple, fish, rain, pen, water, smile, talk, life, sky.

If you cannot asleep

- Think of three different words, any words which just come to your mind at the moment and make a simple story using these 3 words. Repeat untill you fall asleep.

If above does not help

- Stand up and go to the toilet (when possible with as little light as possible)
- Say slowly whenever you are invaded by the thoughts about eating: sun, flower, seven, path, tee, run, yellow, apple, fish, rain, pen, water, smile, talk, life, sky.
- Think of three different words, any words which just come to your mind at the moment and make a simple story using these 3 words. Repeat untill you fall asleep.

If above does not help

- Say STOP untill you fall asleep

If above does not help

- Go to the kitchen and have a very small snack.
- Back to the bed think of three different words, any words which just come to your mind at the moment and make a simple story using these 3 words. Repeat untill you fall asleep.
- If above does not help think of three different words, any words which just come to your mind at the moment and make a simple story using these 3 words. Repeat untill you fall asleep.
- Say slowly whenever you are invaded by the thoughts about eating: sun, flower, seven, path, tee, run, yellow, apple, fish, rain, pen, water, smile, talk, life, sky. Repeat untill you fall asleep.

***

Day 2

Morning

* Say STOP whenever thoughts about eating come to your mind.

* Say slowly whenever you are invaded by the thoughts about eating: sun, flower, seven, path, tee, run, yellow, apple, fish, rain, pen, water, smile, talk, life, sky.

* If above does not help to stop the thoughts about eating just turn your attention away from the invading thoughts about eating. The best way to turn your attention away from the invading thoughts about eating in your head is by doing one of your favorite occupations. Do not be ashamed of any occupation to turn your attention away from the invading thoughts in your head. ALWAYS be busy with your favorite occupation when unsupportable thoughts come to your head.

* Be careful to keep for yourself these of your believes which are found to be strange by the people.

* CONTROL what you say. Say only things which are not strange for the people. You surely already know which of your believes are found to be strange by the people.

* If you do not know yet which of your believes are found to be strange by the people, OBSERVE how people react on what you say. If you see that people are ALERTED by your believes, it means your believes are strange. From now on AVOID presenting such believes.

* Think of three different words, any words which just come to your mind at the moment and make a simple story using these 3 words. Repeat 3 times.

* Try to concentrate on an object close to you, any object. What do you feel when looking at the object? What thoughts come to your mind when looking at the object? And why? Maybe there is a reason. Look for the reason but not too long. If you don't find the reason, forget it.

* Small physical excercise (10 min)

* Small breakfast.

* Nice talk (no complaints, no problematic questions) 10 min. When nobody to talk with, phone or internet conversation oral or written.

* Walk 15 min.

* If you have invading thoughts about eating, ask yourself if it is possible to ignore them.

Yes

Great! In such a case continue ignoring them.

No

You have to learn to ignore the invading thoughts about eating.

This Guide will teach you to ignore the invading thoughts about eating.

Remember: even if you cannot stop the invading thoughts, the invading thoughts cannot stop you to live a normal life.

If you believe in things which other people consider strange, try to keep your strange believes for yourself. Everybody has to make the selection of what can be told to other people and what must be private. Believe me, many people have strange believes. Even much stranger than yours. And they are not considered to be sick. Why? Because they keep their strange believes for themselves. That is the secret.

***

Afternoon

* Say slowly whenever you are invaded by the thoughts about eating: sun, flower, seven, path, tee, run, yellow, apple, fish, rain, pen, water, smile, talk, life, sky.

* Think of three different words, any words which just come to your mind at the moment and make a simple story using these 3 words. Repeat 3 times.

* Try to concentrate on an object close to you, any object. What do you feel when looking at the object? What thoughts come to your mind when looking at the

object? And why? Maybe there is a reason. Look for the reason but not too long. If you don't find the reason, forget it.

* Dinner and half an hour break (you can sleep).

* Nice talk (no complaints) 15 min. When nobody to talk with, phone or internet conversation oral or written.

* Walk 20 min.

* If you have the invading thoughts about eating, ask yourself if it is possible to ignore them.

Yes

Great! In such a case continue ignoring them.

No

You have to learn to ignore the invading thoughts.

This Guide will teach you to ignore the invading thoughts about eating.

Remember: even if you cannot stop the invading thoughts, the invading thoughts cannot stop you to live a normal life.

If you believe in things which other people consider strange, try to keep your strange believes for yourself. Everybody has to make the selection of what can be

told to other people and what must be private. Believe me, many people have strange believes. Even much stranger than yours. And they are not considered to be sick. Why? Because they keep their strange believes for themselves. That is the secret.

***

Evening

- Say slowly whenever you are invaded by the thoughts about eating: sun, flower, seven, path, tee, run, yellow, apple, fish, rain, pen, water, smile, talk, life, sky.

- Think of three different words, any words which just come to your mind at the moment and make a simple story using these 3 words. Repeat 3 times.
  - Try to concentrate on an object close to you, any object. What do you feel when looking at the object? What thoughts come to your mind when looking at the object? And why? Maybe there is a reason. Look for the reason but not too long. If you don't find the reason, forget it.
  - Small supper.
  - Nice talk (no complaints) 10 min. When nobody to talk with, phone or internet conversation oral or written.

- Walk 10 min.
- If you have the invading thoughts about eating, ask yourself if it is possible to ignore them.

Yes

Great! In such a case continue ignoring them.

No

You have to learn to ignore the invading thoughts.

This Guide will teach you to ignore the invading thoughts.

Remember: even if you cannot stop the invading thoughts, the invading thoughts cannot stop you to live a normal life.

If you believe in things which other people consider strange, try to keep your strange believes for yourself. Everybody has to make the selection of what can be told to other people and what must be private. Believe me, many people have strange believes. Even much stranger than yours. And they are not considered to be sick. Why? Because they keep their strange believes for themselves. That is the secret.

***

Night

Before sleep

- Take a shower (warm water) 1 min.
- Small physical excercise 3 min.

In Bed

- Repeat STOP (10 times if you have invading thoughts).
- Say slowly whenever you are invaded by the thoughts about eating: sun, flower, seven, path, tee, run, yellow, apple, fish, rain, pen, water, smile, talk, life, sky.
- Think of three different words, any words which just come to your mind at the moment and make a simple story using these 3 words. Repeat untill you fall asleep.

If you cannot fall asleep

- Say slowly whenever you are invaded by the thoughts about eating: sun, flower, seven, path, tee, run, yellow, apple, fish, rain, pen, water, smile, talk, life, sky.

If you cannot asleep

- Think of three different words, any words which just come to your mind at the moment and make a simple story using these 3 words. Repeat untill you fall asleep.

If above does not help

- Stand up and go to the toilet (when possible with as little light as possible)
- Say slowly whenever you are invaded by the thoughts about eating: sun, flower, seven, path, tee, run, yellow, apple, fish, rain, pen, water, smile, talk, life, sky.
- Think of three different words, any words which just come to your mind at the moment and make a simple story using these 3 words. Repeat untill you fall asleep.

If above does not help

- Say STOP untill you fall asleep

If above does not help

- Go to the kitchen and have a very small snack.
- Back to the bed think of three different words, any words which just come to your mind at the moment and make a simple story using these 3 words. Repeat untill you fall asleep.
- If above does not help think of three different words, any words which just come to your mind at the moment and make a simple story using these 3 words. Repeat untill you fall asleep.

- Say slowly whenever you are invaded by the thoughts about eating: sun, flower, seven, path, tee, run, yellow, apple, fish, rain, pen, water, smile, talk, life, sky. Repeat untill you fall asleep.

***

Day 3

Morning

* Say STOP whenever thoughts about eating come to your mind.

* Say slowly whenever you are invaded by the thoughts about eating: sun, flower, seven, path, tee, run, yellow, apple, fish, rain, pen, water, smile, talk, life, sky.

* If above does not help to stop the thoughts about eating just turn your attention away from the invading thoughts about eating. The best way to turn your attention away from the invading thoughts about eating in your head is by doing one of your favorite occupations. Do not be ashamed of any occupation to turn your attention away from the invading thoughts in your head. ALWAYS be busy with your favorite occupation when unsupportable thoughts come to your head.

* Be careful to keep for yourself these of your believes which are found to be strange by the people.

* CONTROL what you say. Say only things which are not strange for the people. You surely already know which of your believes are found to be strange by the people.

* If you do not know yet which of your believes are found to be strange by the people, OBSERVE how people react on what you say. If you see that people are ALERTED by your believes, it means your believes are strange. From now on AVOID presenting such believes.

* Think of three different words, any words which just come to your mind at the moment and make a simple story using these 3 words. Repeat 3 times.

* Try to concentrate on an object close to you, any object. What do you feel when looking at the object? What thoughts come to your mind when looking at the object? And why? Maybe there is a reason. Look for the reason but not too long. If you don't find the reason, forget it.

* Small physical excercise (10 min)

* Small breakfast.

* Nice talk (no complaints, no problematic questions) 10 min. When nobody to talk with, phone or internet conversation oral or written.

* Walk 15 min.

* If you have invading thoughts about eating, ask yourself if it is possible to ignore them.

Yes

Great! In such a case continue ignoring them.

No

You have to learn to ignore the invading thoughts about eating.

This Guide will teach you to ignore the invading thoughts about eating.

Remember: even if you cannot stop the invading thoughts, the invading thoughts cannot stop you to live a normal life.

If you believe in things which other people consider strange, try to keep your strange believes for yourself. Everybody has to make the selection of what can be told to other people and what must be private. Believe me, many people have strange believes. Even much stranger than yours. And they are not considered to be

sick. Why? Because they keep their strange believes for themselves. That is the secret.

***

Afternoon

* Say slowly whenever you are invaded by the thoughts about eating: sun, flower, seven, path, tee, run, yellow, apple, fish, rain, pen, water, smile, talk, life, sky.

* Think of three different words, any words which just come to your mind at the moment and make a simple story using these 3 words. Repeat 3 times.

* Try to concentrate on an object close to you, any object. What do you feel when looking at the object? What thoughts come to your mind when looking at the object? And why? Maybe there is a reason. Look for the reason but not too long. If you don't find the reason, forget it.

* Dinner and half an hour break (you can sleep).

* Nice talk (no complaints) 15 min. When nobody to talk with, phone or internet conversation oral or written.

* Walk 20 min.

* If you have the invading thoughts about eating, ask yourself if it is possible to ignore them.

Yes

Great! In such a case continue ignoring them.

No

You have to learn to ignore the invading thoughts.

This Guide will teach you to ignore the invading thoughts about eating.

Remember: even if you cannot stop the invading thoughts, the invading thoughts cannot stop you to live a normal life.

If you believe in things which other people consider strange, try to keep your strange believes for yourself. Everybody has to make the selection of what can be told to other people and what must be private. Believe me, many people have strange believes. Even much stranger than yours. And they are not considered to be sick. Why? Because they keep their strange believes for themselves. That is the secret.

***

Evening

- Say slowly whenever you are invaded by the thoughts about eating: sun, flower, seven, path, tee, run, yellow, apple, fish, rain, pen, water, smile, talk, life, sky.

- Think of three different words, any words which just come to your mind at the moment and make a simple story using these 3 words. Repeat 3 times.
  - Try to concentrate on an object close to you, any object. What do you feel when looking at the object? What thoughts come to your mind when looking at the object? And why? Maybe there is a reason. Look for the reason but not too long. If you don't find the reason, forget it.
  - Small supper.
  - Nice talk (no complaints) 10 min. When nobody to talk with, phone or internet conversation oral or written.
  - Walk 10 min.
  - If you have the invading thoughts about eating, ask yourself if it is possible to ignore them.

Yes

Great! In such a case continue ignoring them.

No

You have to learn to ignore the invading thoughts.

This Guide will teach you to ignore the invading thoughts.

Remember: even if you cannot stop the invading thoughts, the invading thoughts cannot stop you to live a normal life.

If you believe in things which other people consider strange, try to keep your strange believes for yourself. Everybody has to make the selection of what can be told to other people and what must be private. Believe me, many people have strange believes. Even much stranger than yours. And they are not considered to be sick. Why? Because they keep their strange believes for themselves. That is the secret.

***

Night

Before sleep

- Take a shower (warm water) 1 min.
- Small physical excercise 3 min.

In Bed

- Repeat STOP (10 times if you have invading thoughts).

- Say slowly whenever you are invaded by the thoughts about eating: sun, flower, seven, path, tee, run, yellow, apple, fish, rain, pen, water, smile, talk, life, sky.
- Think of three different words, any words which just come to your mind at the moment and make a simple story using these 3 words. Repeat untill you fall asleep.

If you cannot fall asleep

- Say slowly whenever you are invaded by the thoughts about eating: sun, flower, seven, path, tee, run, yellow, apple, fish, rain, pen, water, smile, talk, life, sky.

If you cannot asleep

- Think of three different words, any words which just come to your mind at the moment and make a simple story using these 3 words. Repeat untill you fall asleep.

If above does not help

- Stand up and go to the toilet (when possible with as little light as possible)
- Say slowly whenever you are invaded by the thoughts about eating: sun, flower, seven, path,

tee, run, yellow, apple, fish, rain, pen, water, smile, talk, life, sky.
- Think of three different words, any words which just come to your mind at the moment and make a simple story using these 3 words. Repeat untill you fall asleep.

If above does not help

- Say STOP untill you fall asleep

If above does not help

- Go to the kitchen and have a very small snack.
- Back to the bed think of three different words, any words which just come to your mind at the moment and make a simple story using these 3 words. Repeat untill you fall asleep.
- If above does not help think of three different words, any words which just come to your mind at the moment and make a simple story using these 3 words. Repeat untill you fall asleep.
- Say slowly whenever you are invaded by the thoughts about eating: sun, flower, seven, path, tee, run, yellow, apple, fish, rain, pen, water, smile, talk, life, sky. Repeat untill you fall asleep.

***

Day 4

Morning

* Say STOP whenever thoughts about eating come to your mind.

* Say slowly whenever you are invaded by the thoughts about eating: sun, flower, seven, path, tee, run, yellow, apple, fish, rain, pen, water, smile, talk, life, sky.

* If above does not help to stop the thoughts about eating just turn your attention away from the invading thoughts about eating. The best way to turn your attention away from the invading thoughts about eating in your head is by doing one of your favorite occupations. Do not be ashamed of any occupation to turn your attention away from the invading thoughts in your head. ALWAYS be busy with your favorite occupation when unsupportable thoughts come to your head.

* Be careful to keep for yourself these of your believes which are found to be strange by the people.

* CONTROL what you say. Say only things which are not strange for the people. You surely already know which of your believes are found to be strange by the people.

* If you do not know yet which of your believes are found to be strange by the people, OBSERVE how

people react on what you say. If you see that people are ALERTED by your believes, it means your believes are strange. From now on AVOID presenting such believes.

* Think of three different words, any words which just come to your mind at the moment and make a simple story using these 3 words. Repeat 3 times.

* Try to concentrate on an object close to you, any object. What do you feel when looking at the object? What thoughts come to your mind when looking at the object? And why? Maybe there is a reason. Look for the reason but not too long. If you don't find the reason, forget it.

* Small physical excercise (10 min)

* Small breakfast.

* Nice talk (no complaints, no problematic questions) 10 min. When nobody to talk with, phone or internet conversation oral or written.

* Walk 15 min.

* If you have invading thoughts about eating, ask yourself if it is possible to ignore them.

Yes

Great! In such a case continue ignoring them.

No

You have to learn to ignore the invading thoughts about eating.

This Guide will teach you to ignore the invading thoughts about eating.

Remember: even if you cannot stop the invading thoughts, the invading thoughts cannot stop you to live a normal life.

If you believe in things which other people consider strange, try to keep your strange believes for yourself. Everybody has to make the selection of what can be told to other people and what must be private. Believe me, many people have strange believes. Even much stranger than yours. And they are not considered to be sick. Why? Because they keep their strange believes for themselves. That is the secret.

***

Afternoon

* Say slowly whenever you are invaded by the thoughts about eating: sun, flower, seven, path, tee, run, yellow, apple, fish, rain, pen, water, smile, talk, life, sky.

* Think of three different words, any words which just come to your mind at the moment and make a simple story using these 3 words. Repeat 3 times.

* Try to concentrate on an object close to you, any object. What do you feel when looking at the object? What thoughts come to your mind when looking at the object? And why? Maybe there is a reason. Look for the reason but not too long. If you don't find the reason, forget it.

* Dinner and half an hour break (you can sleep).

* Nice talk (no complaints) 15 min. When nobody to talk with, phone or internet conversation oral or written.

* Walk 20 min.

* If you have the invading thoughts about eating, ask yourself if it is possible to ignore them.

Yes

Great! In such a case continue ignoring them.

No

You have to learn to ignore the invading thoughts.

This Guide will teach you to ignore the invading thoughts about eating.

Remember: even if you cannot stop the invading thoughts, the invading thoughts cannot stop you to live a normal life.

If you believe in things which other people consider strange, try to keep your strange believes for yourself. Everybody has to make the selection of what can be told to other people and what must be private. Believe me, many people have strange believes. Even much stranger than yours. And they are not considered to be sick. Why? Because they keep their strange believes for themselves. That is the secret.

***

Evening

- Say slowly whenever you are invaded by the thoughts about eating: sun, flower, seven, path, tee, run, yellow, apple, fish, rain, pen, water, smile, talk, life, sky.

- Think of three different words, any words which just come to your mind at the moment and make a simple story using these 3 words. Repeat 3 times.
  - Try to concentrate on an object close to you, any object. What do you feel when looking at the object? What thoughts come to your mind when

looking at the object? And why? Maybe there is a reason. Look for the reason but not too long. If you don't find the reason, forget it.

- Small supper.
- Nice talk (no complaints) 10 min. When nobody to talk with, phone or internet conversation oral or written.
- Walk 10 min.
- If you have the invading thoughts about eating, ask yourself if it is possible to ignore them.

Yes

Great! In such a case continue ignoring them.

No

You have to learn to ignore the invading thoughts.

This Guide will teach you to ignore the invading thoughts.

Remember: even if you cannot stop the invading thoughts, the invading thoughts cannot stop you to live a normal life.

If you believe in things which other people consider strange, try to keep your strange believes for yourself. Everybody has to make the selection of what can be told to other people and what must be private. Believe

me, many people have strange believes. Even much stranger than yours. And they are not considered to be sick. Why? Because they keep their strange believes for themselves. That is the secret.

***

Night

Before sleep

- Take a shower (warm water) 1 min.
- Small physical excercise 3 min.

In Bed

- Repeat STOP (10 times if you have invading thoughts).
- Say slowly whenever you are invaded by the thoughts about eating: sun, flower, seven, path, tee, run, yellow, apple, fish, rain, pen, water, smile, talk, life, sky.
- Think of three different words, any words which just come to your mind at the moment and make a simple story using these 3 words. Repeat untill you fall asleep.

If you cannot fall asleep

- Say slowly whenever you are invaded by the thoughts about eating: sun, flower, seven, path,

tee, run, yellow, apple, fish, rain, pen, water, smile, talk, life, sky.

If you cannot asleep

- Think of three different words, any words which just come to your mind at the moment and make a simple story using these 3 words. Repeat untill you fall asleep.

If above does not help

- Stand up and go to the toilet (when possible with as little light as possible)
- Say slowly whenever you are invaded by the thoughts about eating: sun, flower, seven, path, tee, run, yellow, apple, fish, rain, pen, water, smile, talk, life, sky.
- Think of three different words, any words which just come to your mind at the moment and make a simple story using these 3 words. Repeat untill you fall asleep.

If above does not help

- Say STOP untill you fall asleep

If above does not help

- Go to the kitchen and have a very small snack.

- Back to the bed think of three different words, any words which just come to your mind at the moment and make a simple story using these 3 words. Repeat untill you fall asleep.
- If above does not help think of three different words, any words which just come to your mind at the moment and make a simple story using these 3 words. Repeat untill you fall asleep.
- Say slowly whenever you are invaded by the thoughts about eating: sun, flower, seven, path, tee, run, yellow, apple, fish, rain, pen, water, smile, talk, life, sky. Repeat untill you fall asleep.

***

Day 5

Morning

* Say STOP whenever thoughts about eating come to your mind.

* Say slowly whenever you are invaded by the thoughts about eating: sun, flower, seven, path, tee, run, yellow, apple, fish, rain, pen, water, smile, talk, life, sky.

* If above does not help to stop the thoughts about eating just turn your attention away from the invading thoughts about eating. The best way to turn your

attention away from the invading thoughts about eating in your head is by doing one of your favorite occupations. Do not be ashamed of any occupation to turn your attention away from the invading thoughts in your head. ALWAYS be busy with your favorite occupation when unsupportable thoughts come to your head.

* Be careful to keep for yourself these of your believes which are found to be strange by the people.

* CONTROL what you say. Say only things which are not strange for the people. You surely already know which of your believes are found to be strange by the people.

* If you do not know yet which of your believes are found to be strange by the people, OBSERVE how people react on what you say. If you see that people are ALERTED by your believes, it means your believes are strange. From now on AVOID presenting such believes.

* Think of three different words, any words which just come to your mind at the moment and make a simple story using these 3 words. Repeat 3 times.

* Try to concentrate on an object close to you, any object. What do you feel when looking at the object? What thoughts come to your mind when looking at the object? And why?Maybe there is a reason. Look for the

reason but not too long. If you don't find the reason, forget it.

* Small physical excercise (10 min)

* Small breakfast.

* Nice talk (no complaints, no problematic questions) 10 min. When nobody to talk with, phone or internet conversation oral or written.

* Walk 15 min.

* If you have invading thoughts about eating, ask yourself if it is possible to ignore them.

Yes

Great! In such a case continue ignoring them.

No

You have to learn to ignore the invading thoughts about eating.

This Guide will teach you to ignore the invading thoughts about eating.

Remember: even if you cannot stop the invading thoughts, the invading thoughts cannot stop you to live a normal life.

If you believe in things which other people consider strange, try to keep your strange believes for yourself. Everybody has to make the selection of what can be told to other people and what must be private. Believe me, many people have strange believes. Even much stranger than yours. And they are not considered to be sick. Why? Because they keep their strange believes for themselves. That is the secret.

***

Afternoon

* Say slowly whenever you are invaded by the thoughts about eating: sun, flower, seven, path, tee, run, yellow, apple, fish, rain, pen, water, smile, talk, life, sky.

* Think of three different words, any words which just come to your mind at the moment and make a simple story using these 3 words. Repeat 3 times.

* Try to concentrate on an object close to you, any object. What do you feel when looking at the object? What thoughts come to your mind when looking at the object? And why? Maybe there is a reason. Look for the reason but not too long. If you don't find the reason, forget it.

* Dinner and half an hour break (you can sleep).

* Nice talk (no complaints) 15 min. When nobody to talk with, phone or internet conversation oral or written.

* Walk 20 min.

* If you have the invading thoughts about eating, ask yourself if it is possible to ignore them.

Yes

Great! In such a case continue ignoring them.

No

You have to learn to ignore the invading thoughts.

This Guide will teach you to ignore the invading thoughts about eating.

Remember: even if you cannot stop the invading thoughts, the invading thoughts cannot stop you to live a normal life.

If you believe in things which other people consider strange, try to keep your strange believes for yourself. Everybody has to make the selection of what can be told to other people and what must be private. Believe me, many people have strange believes. Even much stranger than yours. And they are not considered to be

sick. Why? Because they keep their strange believes for themselves. That is the secret.

***

Evening

- Say slowly whenever you are invaded by the thoughts about eating: sun, flower, seven, path, tee, run, yellow, apple, fish, rain, pen, water, smile, talk, life, sky.

- Think of three different words, any words which just come to your mind at the moment and make a simple story using these 3 words. Repeat 3 times.
  - Try to concentrate on an object close to you, any object. What do you feel when looking at the object? What thoughts come to your mind when looking at the object? And why? Maybe there is a reason. Look for the reason but not too long. If you don't find the reason, forget it.
  - Small supper.
  - Nice talk (no complaints) 10 min. When nobody to talk with, phone or internet conversation oral or written.
  - Walk 10 min.
  - If you have the invading thoughts about eating, ask yourself if it is possible to ignore them.

Yes

Great! In such a case continue ignoring them.

No

You have to learn to ignore the invading thoughts.

This Guide will teach you to ignore the invading thoughts.

Remember: even if you cannot stop the invading thoughts, the invading thoughts cannot stop you to live a normal life.

If you believe in things which other people consider strange, try to keep your strange believes for yourself. Everybody has to make the selection of what can be told to other people and what must be private. Believe me, many people have strange believes. Even much stranger than yours. And they are not considered to be sick. Why? Because they keep their strange believes for themselves. That is the secret.

***

Night

Before sleep

- Take a shower (warm water) 1 min.
- Small physical excercise 3 min.

In Bed

- Repeat STOP (10 times if you have invading thoughts).
- Say slowly whenever you are invaded by the thoughts about eating: sun, flower, seven, path, tee, run, yellow, apple, fish, rain, pen, water, smile, talk, life, sky.
- Think of three different words, any words which just come to your mind at the moment and make a simple story using these 3 words. Repeat untill you fall asleep.

If you cannot fall asleep

- Say slowly whenever you are invaded by the thoughts about eating: sun, flower, seven, path, tee, run, yellow, apple, fish, rain, pen, water, smile, talk, life, sky.

If you cannot asleep

- Think of three different words, any words which just come to your mind at the moment and make a simple story using these 3 words. Repeat untill you fall asleep.

If above does not help

- Stand up and go to the toilet (when possible with as little light as possible)

- Say slowly whenever you are invaded by the thoughts about eating: sun, flower, seven, path, tee, run, yellow, apple, fish, rain, pen, water, smile, talk, life, sky.
- Think of three different words, any words which just come to your mind at the moment and make a simple story using these 3 words. Repeat untill you fall asleep.

If above does not help

- Say STOP untill you fall asleep

If above does not help

- Go to the kitchen and have a very small snack.
- Back to the bed think of three different words, any words which just come to your mind at the moment and make a simple story using these 3 words. Repeat untill you fall asleep.
- If above does not help think of three different words, any words which just come to your mind at the moment and make a simple story using these 3 words. Repeat untill you fall asleep.
- Say slowly whenever you are invaded by the thoughts about eating: sun, flower, seven, path, tee, run, yellow, apple, fish, rain, pen, water, smile, talk, life, sky. Repeat untill you fall asleep.

***

Day 6

Morning

* Say STOP whenever thoughts about eating come to your mind.

* Say slowly whenever you are invaded by the thoughts about eating: sun, flower, seven, path, tee, run, yellow, apple, fish, rain, pen, water, smile, talk, life, sky.

* If above does not help to stop the thoughts about eating just turn your attention away from the invading thoughts about eating. The best way to turn your attention away from the invading thoughts about eating in your head is by doing one of your favorite occupations. Do not be ashamed of any occupation to turn your attention away from the invading thoughts in your head. ALWAYS be busy with your favorite occupation when unsupportable thoughts come to your head.

* Be careful to keep for yourself these of your believes which are found to be strange by the people.

* CONTROL what you say. Say only things which are not strange for the people. You surely already know which of your believes are found to be strange by the people.

* If you do not know yet which of your believes are found to be strange by the people, OBSERVE how people react on what you say. If you see that people are ALERTED by your believes, it means your believes are strange. From now on AVOID presenting such believes.

* Think of three different words, any words which just come to your mind at the moment and make a simple story using these 3 words. Repeat 3 times.

* Try to concentrate on an object close to you, any object. What do you feel when looking at the object? What thoughts come to your mind when looking at the object? And why? Maybe there is a reason. Look for the reason but not too long. If you don't find the reason, forget it.

* Small physical excercise (10 min)

* Small breakfast.

* Nice talk (no complaints, no problematic questions) 10 min. When nobody to talk with, phone or internet conversation oral or written.

* Walk 15 min.

* If you have invading thoughts about eating, ask yourself if it is possible to ignore them.

Yes

Great! In such a case continue ignoring them.

No

You have to learn to ignore the invading thoughts about eating.

This Guide will teach you to ignore the invading thoughts about eating.

Remember: even if you cannot stop the invading thoughts, the invading thoughts cannot stop you to live a normal life.

If you believe in things which other people consider strange, try to keep your strange believes for yourself. Everybody has to make the selection of what can be told to other people and what must be private. Believe me, many people have strange believes. Even much stranger than yours. And they are not considered to be sick. Why? Because they keep their strange believes for themselves. That is the secret.

***

Afternoon

* Say slowly whenever you are invaded by the thoughts about eating: sun, flower, seven, path, tee, run, yellow, apple, fish, rain, pen, water, smile, talk, life, sky.

* Think of three different words, any words which just come to your mind at the moment and make a simple story using these 3 words. Repeat 3 times.

* Try to concentrate on an object close to you, any object. What do you feel when looking at the object? What thoughts come to your mind when looking at the object? And why? Maybe there is a reason. Look for the reason but not too long. If you don't find the reason, forget it.

* Dinner and half an hour break (you can sleep).

* Nice talk (no complaints) 15 min. When nobody to talk with, phone or internet conversation oral or written.

* Walk 20 min.

* If you have the invading thoughts about eating, ask yourself if it is possible to ignore them.

Yes

Great! In such a case continue ignoring them.

No

You have to learn to ignore the invading thoughts.

This Guide will teach you to ignore the invading thoughts about eating.

Remember: even if you cannot stop the invading thoughts, the invading thoughts cannot stop you to live a normal life.

If you believe in things which other people consider strange, try to keep your strange believes for yourself. Everybody has to make the selection of what can be told to other people and what must be private. Believe me, many people have strange believes. Even much stranger than yours. And they are not considered to be sick. Why? Because they keep their strange believes for themselves. That is the secret.

***

Evening

- Say slowly whenever you are invaded by the thoughts about eating: sun, flower, seven, path, tee, run, yellow, apple, fish, rain, pen, water, smile, talk, life, sky.

- Think of three different words, any words which just come to your mind at the moment and make a simple story using these 3 words. Repeat 3 times.

- Try to concentrate on an object close to you, any object. What do you feel when looking at the object? What thoughts come to your mind when looking at the object? And why? Maybe there is a reason. Look for the reason but not too long. If you don't find the reason, forget it.
- Small supper.
- Nice talk (no complaints) 10 min. When nobody to talk with, phone or internet conversation oral or written.
- Walk 10 min.
- If you have the invading thoughts about eating, ask yourself if it is possible to ignore them.

Yes

Great! In such a case continue ignoring them.

No

You have to learn to ignore the invading thoughts.

This Guide will teach you to ignore the invading thoughts.

Remember: even if you cannot stop the invading thoughts, the invading thoughts cannot stop you to live a normal life.

If you believe in things which other people consider strange, try to keep your strange believes for yourself. Everybody has to make the selection of what can be told to other people and what must be private. Believe me, many people have strange believes. Even much stranger than yours. And they are not considered to be sick. Why? Because they keep their strange believes for themselves. That is the secret.

***

Night

Before sleep

- Take a shower (warm water) 1 min.
- Small physical excercise 3 min.

In Bed

- Repeat STOP (10 times if you have invading thoughts).
- Say slowly whenever you are invaded by the thoughts about eating: sun, flower, seven, path, tee, run, yellow, apple, fish, rain, pen, water, smile, talk, life, sky.
- Think of three different words, any words which just come to your mind at the moment and make a simple story using these 3 words. Repeat untill you fall asleep.

If you cannot fall asleep

- Say slowly whenever you are invaded by the thoughts about eating: sun, flower, seven, path, tee, run, yellow, apple, fish, rain, pen, water, smile, talk, life, sky.

If you cannot asleep

- Think of three different words, any words which just come to your mind at the moment and make a simple story using these 3 words. Repeat untill you fall asleep.

If above does not help

- Stand up and go to the toilet (when possible with as little light as possible)
- Say slowly whenever you are invaded by the thoughts about eating: sun, flower, seven, path, tee, run, yellow, apple, fish, rain, pen, water, smile, talk, life, sky.
- Think of three different words, any words which just come to your mind at the moment and make a simple story using these 3 words. Repeat untill you fall asleep.

If above does not help

- Say STOP untill you fall asleep

If above does not help

- Go to the kitchen and have a very small snack.
- Back to the bed think of three different words, any words which just come to your mind at the moment and make a simple story using these 3 words. Repeat untill you fall asleep.
- If above does not help think of three different words, any words which just come to your mind at the moment and make a simple story using these 3 words. Repeat untill you fall asleep.
- Say slowly whenever you are invaded by the thoughts about eating: sun, flower, seven, path, tee, run, yellow, apple, fish, rain, pen, water, smile, talk, life, sky. Repeat untill you fall asleep.

***

Day 7

Morning

* Say STOP whenever thoughts about eating come to your mind.

* Say slowly whenever you are invaded by the thoughts about eating: sun, flower, seven, path, tee, run, yellow, apple, fish, rain, pen, water, smile, talk, life, sky.

* If above does not help to stop the thoughts about eating just turn your attention away from the invading thoughts about eating. The best way to turn your attention away from the invading thoughts about eating in your head is by doing one of your favorite occupations. Do not be ashamed of any occupation to turn your attention away from the invading thoughts in your head. ALWAYS be busy with your favorite occupation when unsupportable thoughts come to your head.

* Be careful to keep for yourself these of your believes which are found to be strange by the people.

* CONTROL what you say. Say only things which are not strange for the people. You surely already know which of your believes are found to be strange by the people.

* If you do not know yet which of your believes are found to be strange by the people, OBSERVE how people react on what you say. If you see that people are ALERTED by your believes, it means your believes are strange. From now on AVOID presenting such believes.

* Think of three different words, any words which just come to your mind at the moment and make a simple story using these 3 words. Repeat 3 times.

* Try to concentrate on an object close to you, any object. What do you feel when looking at the object? What thoughts come to your mind when looking at the object? And why?Maybe there is a reason. Look for the reason but not too long. If you don't find the reason, forget it.

* Small physical excercise (10 min)

* Small breakfast.

* Nice talk (no complaints, no problematic questions) 10 min. When nobody to talk with, phone or internet conversation oral or written.

* Walk 15 min.

* If you have invading thoughts about eating, ask yourself if it is possible to ignore them.

Yes

Great! In such a case continue ignoring them.

No

You have to learn to ignore the invading thoughts about eating.

This Guide will teach you to ignore the invading thoughts about eating.

Remember: even if you cannot stop the invading thoughts, the invading thoughts cannot stop you to live a normal life.

If you believe in things which other people consider strange, try to keep your strange believes for yourself. Everybody has to make the selection of what can be told to other people and what must be private. Believe me, many people have strange believes. Even much stranger than yours. And they are not considered to be sick. Why? Because they keep their strange believes for themselves. That is the secret.

***

Afternoon

* Say slowly whenever you are invaded by the thoughts about eating: sun, flower, seven, path, tee, run, yellow, apple, fish, rain, pen, water, smile, talk, life, sky.

* Think of three different words, any words which just come to your mind at the moment and make a simple story using these 3 words. Repeat 3 times.

* Try to concentrate on an object close to you, any object. What do you feel when looking at the object? What thoughts come to your mind when looking at the

object? And why? Maybe there is a reason. Look for the reason but not too long. If you don't find the reason, forget it.

* Dinner and half an hour break (you can sleep).

* Nice talk (no complaints) 15 min. When nobody to talk with, phone or internet conversation oral or written.

* Walk 20 min.

* If you have the invading thoughts about eating, ask yourself if it is possible to ignore them.

Yes

Great! In such a case continue ignoring them.

No

You have to learn to ignore the invading thoughts.

This Guide will teach you to ignore the invading thoughts about eating.

Remember: even if you cannot stop the invading thoughts, the invading thoughts cannot stop you to live a normal life.

If you believe in things which other people consider strange, try to keep your strange believes for yourself. Everybody has to make the selection of what can be

told to other people and what must be private. Believe me, many people have strange believes. Even much stranger than yours. And they are not considered to be sick. Why? Because they keep their strange believes for themselves. That is the secret.

***

Evening

- Say slowly whenever you are invaded by the thoughts about eating: sun, flower, seven, path, tee, run, yellow, apple, fish, rain, pen, water, smile, talk, life, sky.

- Think of three different words, any words which just come to your mind at the moment and make a simple story using these 3 words. Repeat 3 times.
  - Try to concentrate on an object close to you, any object. What do you feel when looking at the object? What thoughts come to your mind when looking at the object? And why? Maybe there is a reason. Look for the reason but not too long. If you don't find the reason, forget it.
  - Small supper.
  - Nice talk (no complaints) 10 min. When nobody to talk with, phone or internet conversation oral or written.

- Walk 10 min.
- If you have the invading thoughts about eating, ask yourself if it is possible to ignore them.

Yes

Great! In such a case continue ignoring them.

No

You have to learn to ignore the invading thoughts.

This Guide will teach you to ignore the invading thoughts.

Remember: even if you cannot stop the invading thoughts, the invading thoughts cannot stop you to live a normal life.

If you believe in things which other people consider strange, try to keep your strange believes for yourself. Everybody has to make the selection of what can be told to other people and what must be private. Believe me, many people have strange believes. Even much stranger than yours. And they are not considered to be sick. Why? Because they keep their strange believes for themselves. That is the secret.

***

Night

Before sleep

- Take a shower (warm water) 1 min.
- Small physical excercise 3 min.

In Bed

- Repeat STOP (10 times if you have invading thoughts).
- Say slowly whenever you are invaded by the thoughts about eating: sun, flower, seven, path, tee, run, yellow, apple, fish, rain, pen, water, smile, talk, life, sky.
- Think of three different words, any words which just come to your mind at the moment and make a simple story using these 3 words. Repeat untill you fall asleep.

If you cannot fall asleep

- Say slowly whenever you are invaded by the thoughts about eating: sun, flower, seven, path, tee, run, yellow, apple, fish, rain, pen, water, smile, talk, life, sky.

If you cannot asleep

- Think of three different words, any words which just come to your mind at the moment and make a simple story using these 3 words. Repeat untill you fall asleep.

If above does not help

- Stand up and go to the toilet (when possible with as little light as possible)
- Say slowly whenever you are invaded by the thoughts about eating: sun, flower, seven, path, tee, run, yellow, apple, fish, rain, pen, water, smile, talk, life, sky.
- Think of three different words, any words which just come to your mind at the moment and make a simple story using these 3 words. Repeat untill you fall asleep.

If above does not help

- Say STOP untill you fall asleep

If above does not help

- Go to the kitchen and have a very small snack.
- Back to the bed think of three different words, any words which just come to your mind at the moment and make a simple story using these 3 words. Repeat untill you fall asleep.
- If above does not help think of three different words, any words which just come to your mind at the moment and make a simple story using these 3 words. Repeat untill you fall asleep.

- Say slowly whenever you are invaded by the thoughts about eating: sun, flower, seven, path, tee, run, yellow, apple, fish, rain, pen, water, smile, talk, life, sky. Repeat untill you fall asleep.

***

Week Seven

Day 1

Morning

* Say STOP whenever thoughts about eating come to your mind.

* Say slowly whenever you are invaded by the thoughts about eating: sun, flower, seven, path, tee, run, yellow, apple, fish, rain, pen, water, smile, talk, life, sky.

* If above does not help to stop the thoughts about eating just turn your attention away from the invading thoughts about eating. The best way to turn your attention away from the invading thoughts about eating in your head is by doing one of your favorite occupations. Do not be ashamed of any occupation to turn your attention away from the invading thoughts in your head. ALWAYS be busy with your favorite occupation when unsupportable thoughts come to your head.

* Be careful to keep for yourself these of your believes which are found to be strange by the people.

* CONTROL what you say. Say only things which are not strange for the people. You surely already know which of your believes are found to be strange by the people.

* If you do not know yet which of your believes are found to be strange by the people, OBSERVE how people react on what you say. If you see that people are ALERTED by your believes, it means your believes are strange. From now on AVOID presenting such believes.

* Think of three different words, any words which just come to your mind at the moment and make a simple story using these 3 words. Repeat 3 times.

* Try to concentrate on an object close to you, any object. What do you feel when looking at the object? What thoughts come to your mind when looking at the object? And why?Maybe there is a reason. Look for the reason but not too long. If you don't find the reason, forget it.

* Small physical excercise (10 min)

* Small breakfast.

* Nice talk (no complaints, no problematic questions) 10 min. When nobody to talk with, phone or internet conversation oral or written.

* Walk 15 min.

* If you have invading thoughts about eating, ask yourself if it is possible to ignore them.

Yes

Great! In such a case continue ignoring them.

No

You have to learn to ignore the invading thoughts about eating.

This Guide will teach you to ignore the invading thoughts about eating.

Remember: even if you cannot stop the invading thoughts, the invading thoughts cannot stop you to live a normal life.

If you believe in things which other people consider strange, try to keep your strange believes for yourself. Everybody has to make the selection of what can be told to other people and what must be private. Believe me, many people have strange believes. Even much stranger than yours. And they are not considered to be

sick. Why? Because they keep their strange believes for themselves. That is the secret.

***

Afternoon

* Say slowly whenever you are invaded by the thoughts about eating: sun, flower, seven, path, tee, run, yellow, apple, fish, rain, pen, water, smile, talk, life, sky.

* Think of three different words, any words which just come to your mind at the moment and make a simple story using these 3 words. Repeat 3 times.

* Try to concentrate on an object close to you, any object. What do you feel when looking at the object? What thoughts come to your mind when looking at the object? And why?Maybe there is a reason. Look for the reason but not too long. If you don't find the reason, forget it.

* Dinner and half an hour break (you can sleep).

* Nice talk (no complaints) 15 min. When nobody to talk with, phone or internet conversation oral or written.

* Walk 20 min.

* If you have the invading thoughts about eating, ask yourself if it is possible to ignore them.

Yes

Great! In such a case continue ignoring them.

No

You have to learn to ignore the invading thoughts.

This Guide will teach you to ignore the invading thoughts about eating.

Remember: even if you cannot stop the invading thoughts, the invading thoughts cannot stop you to live a normal life.

If you believe in things which other people consider strange, try to keep your strange believes for yourself. Everybody has to make the selection of what can be told to other people and what must be private. Believe me, many people have strange believes. Even much stranger than yours. And they are not considered to be sick. Why? Because they keep their strange believes for themselves. That is the secret.

***

Evening

- Say slowly whenever you are invaded by the thoughts about eating: sun, flower, seven, path, tee, run, yellow, apple, fish, rain, pen, water, smile, talk, life, sky.

- Think of three different words, any words which just come to your mind at the moment and make a simple story using these 3 words. Repeat 3 times.
  - Try to concentrate on an object close to you, any object. What do you feel when looking at the object? What thoughts come to your mind when looking at the object? And why? Maybe there is a reason. Look for the reason but not too long. If you don't find the reason, forget it.
  - Small supper.
  - Nice talk (no complaints) 10 min. When nobody to talk with, phone or internet conversation oral or written.
  - Walk 10 min.
  - If you have the invading thoughts about eating, ask yourself if it is possible to ignore them.

Yes

Great! In such a case continue ignoring them.

No

You have to learn to ignore the invading thoughts.

This Guide will teach you to ignore the invading thoughts.

Remember: even if you cannot stop the invading thoughts, the invading thoughts cannot stop you to live a normal life.

If you believe in things which other people consider strange, try to keep your strange believes for yourself. Everybody has to make the selection of what can be told to other people and what must be private. Believe me, many people have strange believes. Even much stranger than yours. And they are not considered to be sick. Why? Because they keep their strange believes for themselves. That is the secret.

***

Night

Before sleep

- Take a shower (warm water) 1 min.
- Small physical excercise 3 min.

In Bed

- Repeat STOP (10 times if you have invading thoughts).

- Say slowly whenever you are invaded by the thoughts about eating: sun, flower, seven, path, tee, run, yellow, apple, fish, rain, pen, water, smile, talk, life, sky.
- Think of three different words, any words which just come to your mind at the moment and make a simple story using these 3 words. Repeat untill you fall asleep.

If you cannot fall asleep

- Say slowly whenever you are invaded by the thoughts about eating: sun, flower, seven, path, tee, run, yellow, apple, fish, rain, pen, water, smile, talk, life, sky.

If you cannot asleep

- Think of three different words, any words which just come to your mind at the moment and make a simple story using these 3 words. Repeat untill you fall asleep.

If above does not help

- Stand up and go to the toilet (when possible with as little light as possible)
- Say slowly whenever you are invaded by the thoughts about eating: sun, flower, seven, path,

tee, run, yellow, apple, fish, rain, pen, water, smile, talk, life, sky.
- Think of three different words, any words which just come to your mind at the moment and make a simple story using these 3 words. Repeat untill you fall asleep.

If above does not help
- Say STOP untill you fall asleep

If above does not help
- Go to the kitchen and have a very small snack.
- Back to the bed think of three different words, any words which just come to your mind at the moment and make a simple story using these 3 words. Repeat untill you fall asleep.
- If above does not help think of three different words, any words which just come to your mind at the moment and make a simple story using these 3 words. Repeat untill you fall asleep.
- Say slowly whenever you are invaded by the thoughts about eating: sun, flower, seven, path, tee, run, yellow, apple, fish, rain, pen, water, smile, talk, life, sky. Repeat untill you fall asleep.

***

Day 2

Morning

* Say STOP whenever thoughts about eating come to your mind.

* Say slowly whenever you are invaded by the thoughts about eating: sun, flower, seven, path, tee, run, yellow, apple, fish, rain, pen, water, smile, talk, life, sky.

* If above does not help to stop the thoughts about eating just turn your attention away from the invading thoughts about eating. The best way to turn your attention away from the invading thoughts about eating in your head is by doing one of your favorite occupations. Do not be ashamed of any occupation to turn your attention away from the invading thoughts in your head. ALWAYS be busy with your favorite occupation when unsupportable thoughts come to your head.

* Be careful to keep for yourself these of your believes which are found to be strange by the people.

* CONTROL what you say. Say only things which are not strange for the people. You surely already know which of your believes are found to be strange by the people.

* If you do not know yet which of your believes are found to be strange by the people, OBSERVE how

people react on what you say. If you see that people are ALERTED by your believes, it means your believes are strange. From now on AVOID presenting such believes.

* Think of three different words, any words which just come to your mind at the moment and make a simple story using these 3 words. Repeat 3 times.

* Try to concentrate on an object close to you, any object. What do you feel when looking at the object? What thoughts come to your mind when looking at the object? And why?Maybe there is a reason. Look for the reason but not too long. If you don't find the reason, forget it.

* Small physical excercise (10 min)

* Small breakfast.

* Nice talk (no complaints, no problematic questions) 10 min. When nobody to talk with, phone or internet conversation oral or written.

* Walk 15 min.

* If you have invading thoughts about eating, ask yourself if it is possible to ignore them.

Yes

Great! In such a case continue ignoring them.

No

You have to learn to ignore the invading thoughts about eating.

This Guide will teach you to ignore the invading thoughts about eating.

Remember: even if you cannot stop the invading thoughts, the invading thoughts cannot stop you to live a normal life.

If you believe in things which other people consider strange, try to keep your strange believes for yourself. Everybody has to make the selection of what can be told to other people and what must be private. Believe me, many people have strange believes. Even much stranger than yours. And they are not considered to be sick. Why? Because they keep their strange believes for themselves. That is the secret.

***

Afternoon

* Say slowly whenever you are invaded by the thoughts about eating: sun, flower, seven, path, tee, run, yellow, apple, fish, rain, pen, water, smile, talk, life, sky.

* Think of three different words, any words which just come to your mind at the moment and make a simple story using these 3 words. Repeat 3 times.

* Try to concentrate on an object close to you, any object. What do you feel when looking at the object? What thoughts come to your mind when looking at the object? And why? Maybe there is a reason. Look for the reason but not too long. If you don't find the reason, forget it.

* Dinner and half an hour break (you can sleep).

* Nice talk (no complaints) 15 min. When nobody to talk with, phone or internet conversation oral or written.

* Walk 20 min.

* If you have the invading thoughts about eating, ask yourself if it is possible to ignore them.

Yes

Great! In such a case continue ignoring them.

No

You have to learn to ignore the invading thoughts.

This Guide will teach you to ignore the invading thoughts about eating.

Remember: even if you cannot stop the invading thoughts, the invading thoughts cannot stop you to live a normal life.

If you believe in things which other people consider strange, try to keep your strange believes for yourself. Everybody has to make the selection of what can be told to other people and what must be private. Believe me, many people have strange believes. Even much stranger than yours. And they are not considered to be sick. Why? Because they keep their strange believes for themselves. That is the secret.

***

Evening

- Say slowly whenever you are invaded by the thoughts about eating: sun, flower, seven, path, tee, run, yellow, apple, fish, rain, pen, water, smile, talk, life, sky.

- Think of three different words, any words which just come to your mind at the moment and make a simple story using these 3 words. Repeat 3 times.
  - Try to concentrate on an object close to you, any object. What do you feel when looking at the object? What thoughts come to your mind when

looking at the object? And why? Maybe there is a reason. Look for the reason but not too long. If you don't find the reason, forget it.

- Small supper.
- Nice talk (no complaints) 10 min. When nobody to talk with, phone or internet conversation oral or written.
- Walk 10 min.
- If you have the invading thoughts about eating, ask yourself if it is possible to ignore them.

Yes

Great! In such a case continue ignoring them.

No

You have to learn to ignore the invading thoughts.

This Guide will teach you to ignore the invading thoughts.

Remember: even if you cannot stop the invading thoughts, the invading thoughts cannot stop you to live a normal life.

If you believe in things which other people consider strange, try to keep your strange believes for yourself. Everybody has to make the selection of what can be told to other people and what must be private. Believe

me, many people have strange believes. Even much stranger than yours. And they are not considered to be sick. Why? Because they keep their strange believes for themselves. That is the secret.

***

Night

Before sleep

- Take a shower (warm water) 1 min.
- Small physical excercise 3 min.

In Bed

- Repeat STOP (10 times if you have invading thoughts).
- Say slowly whenever you are invaded by the thoughts about eating: sun, flower, seven, path, tee, run, yellow, apple, fish, rain, pen, water, smile, talk, life, sky.
- Think of three different words, any words which just come to your mind at the moment and make a simple story using these 3 words. Repeat untill you fall asleep.

If you cannot fall asleep

- Say slowly whenever you are invaded by the thoughts about eating: sun, flower, seven, path,

tee, run, yellow, apple, fish, rain, pen, water, smile, talk, life, sky.

If you cannot asleep

- Think of three different words, any words which just come to your mind at the moment and make a simple story using these 3 words. Repeat untill you fall asleep.

If above does not help

- Stand up and go to the toilet (when possible with as little light as possible)
- Say slowly whenever you are invaded by the thoughts about eating: sun, flower, seven, path, tee, run, yellow, apple, fish, rain, pen, water, smile, talk, life, sky.
- Think of three different words, any words which just come to your mind at the moment and make a simple story using these 3 words. Repeat untill you fall asleep.

If above does not help

- Say STOP untill you fall asleep

If above does not help

- Go to the kitchen and have a very small snack.

- Back to the bed think of three different words, any words which just come to your mind at the moment and make a simple story using these 3 words. Repeat untill you fall asleep.
- If above does not help think of three different words, any words which just come to your mind at the moment and make a simple story using these 3 words. Repeat untill you fall asleep.
- Say slowly whenever you are invaded by the thoughts about eating: sun, flower, seven, path, tee, run, yellow, apple, fish, rain, pen, water, smile, talk, life, sky. Repeat untill you fall asleep.

***

Day 3

Morning

* Say STOP whenever thoughts about eating come to your mind.

* Say slowly whenever you are invaded by the thoughts about eating: sun, flower, seven, path, tee, run, yellow, apple, fish, rain, pen, water, smile, talk, life, sky.

* If above does not help to stop the thoughts about eating just turn your attention away from the invading thoughts about eating. The best way to turn your

attention away from the invading thoughts about eating in your head is by doing one of your favorite occupations. Do not be ashamed of any occupation to turn your attention away from the invading thoughts in your head. ALWAYS be busy with your favorite occupation when unsupportable thoughts come to your head.

* Be careful to keep for yourself these of your believes which are found to be strange by the people.

* CONTROL what you say. Say only things which are not strange for the people. You surely already know which of your believes are found to be strange by the people.

* If you do not know yet which of your believes are found to be strange by the people, OBSERVE how people react on what you say. If you see that people are ALERTED by your believes, it means your believes are strange. From now on AVOID presenting such believes.

* Think of three different words, any words which just come to your mind at the moment and make a simple story using these 3 words. Repeat 3 times.

* Try to concentrate on an object close to you, any object. What do you feel when looking at the object? What thoughts come to your mind when looking at the object? And why?Maybe there is a reason. Look for the

reason but not too long. If you don't find the reason, forget it.

* Small physical excercise (10 min)

* Small breakfast.

* Nice talk (no complaints, no problematic questions) 10 min. When nobody to talk with, phone or internet conversation oral or written.

* Walk 15 min.

* If you have invading thoughts about eating, ask yourself if it is possible to ignore them.

Yes

Great! In such a case continue ignoring them.

No

You have to learn to ignore the invading thoughts about eating.

This Guide will teach you to ignore the invading thoughts about eating.

Remember: even if you cannot stop the invading thoughts, the invading thoughts cannot stop you to live a normal life.

If you believe in things which other people consider strange, try to keep your strange believes for yourself. Everybody has to make the selection of what can be told to other people and what must be private. Believe me, many people have strange believes. Even much stranger than yours. And they are not considered to be sick. Why? Because they keep their strange believes for themselves. That is the secret.

***

Afternoon

* Say slowly whenever you are invaded by the thoughts about eating: sun, flower, seven, path, tee, run, yellow, apple, fish, rain, pen, water, smile, talk, life, sky.

* Think of three different words, any words which just come to your mind at the moment and make a simple story using these 3 words. Repeat 3 times.

* Try to concentrate on an object close to you, any object. What do you feel when looking at the object? What thoughts come to your mind when looking at the object? And why? Maybe there is a reason. Look for the reason but not too long. If you don't find the reason, forget it.

* Dinner and half an hour break (you can sleep).

* Nice talk (no complaints) 15 min. When nobody to talk with, phone or internet conversation oral or written.

* Walk 20 min.

* If you have the invading thoughts about eating, ask yourself if it is possible to ignore them.

Yes

Great! In such a case continue ignoring them.

No

You have to learn to ignore the invading thoughts.

This Guide will teach you to ignore the invading thoughts about eating.

Remember: even if you cannot stop the invading thoughts, the invading thoughts cannot stop you to live a normal life.

If you believe in things which other people consider strange, try to keep your strange believes for yourself. Everybody has to make the selection of what can be told to other people and what must be private. Believe me, many people have strange believes. Even much stranger than yours. And they are not considered to be

sick. Why? Because they keep their strange believes for themselves. That is the secret.

***

Evening

- Say slowly whenever you are invaded by the thoughts about eating: sun, flower, seven, path, tee, run, yellow, apple, fish, rain, pen, water, smile, talk, life, sky.

- Think of three different words, any words which just come to your mind at the moment and make a simple story using these 3 words. Repeat 3 times.
  - Try to concentrate on an object close to you, any object. What do you feel when looking at the object? What thoughts come to your mind when looking at the object? And why? Maybe there is a reason. Look for the reason but not too long. If you don't find the reason, forget it.
  - Small supper.
  - Nice talk (no complaints) 10 min. When nobody to talk with, phone or internet conversation oral or written.
  - Walk 10 min.
  - If you have the invading thoughts about eating, ask yourself if it is possible to ignore them.

Yes

Great! In such a case continue ignoring them.

No

You have to learn to ignore the invading thoughts.

This Guide will teach you to ignore the invading thoughts.

Remember: even if you cannot stop the invading thoughts, the invading thoughts cannot stop you to live a normal life.

If you believe in things which other people consider strange, try to keep your strange believes for yourself. Everybody has to make the selection of what can be told to other people and what must be private. Believe me, many people have strange believes. Even much stranger than yours. And they are not considered to be sick. Why? Because they keep their strange believes for themselves. That is the secret.

***

Night

Before sleep

- Take a shower (warm water) 1 min.
- Small physical excercise 3 min.

In Bed

- Repeat STOP (10 times if you have invading thoughts).
- Say slowly whenever you are invaded by the thoughts about eating: sun, flower, seven, path, tee, run, yellow, apple, fish, rain, pen, water, smile, talk, life, sky.
- Think of three different words, any words which just come to your mind at the moment and make a simple story using these 3 words. Repeat untill you fall asleep.

If you cannot fall asleep

- Say slowly whenever you are invaded by the thoughts about eating: sun, flower, seven, path, tee, run, yellow, apple, fish, rain, pen, water, smile, talk, life, sky.

If you cannot asleep

- Think of three different words, any words which just come to your mind at the moment and make a simple story using these 3 words. Repeat untill you fall asleep.

If above does not help

- Stand up and go to the toilet (when possible with as little light as possible)

- Say slowly whenever you are invaded by the thoughts about eating: sun, flower, seven, path, tee, run, yellow, apple, fish, rain, pen, water, smile, talk, life, sky.
- Think of three different words, any words which just come to your mind at the moment and make a simple story using these 3 words. Repeat untill you fall asleep.

If above does not help

- Say STOP untill you fall asleep

If above does not help

- Go to the kitchen and have a very small snack.
- Back to the bed think of three different words, any words which just come to your mind at the moment and make a simple story using these 3 words. Repeat untill you fall asleep.
- If above does not help think of three different words, any words which just come to your mind at the moment and make a simple story using these 3 words. Repeat untill you fall asleep.
- Say slowly whenever you are invaded by the thoughts about eating: sun, flower, seven, path, tee, run, yellow, apple, fish, rain, pen, water, smile, talk, life, sky. Repeat untill you fall asleep.

***

Day 4

Morning

* Say STOP whenever thoughts about eating come to your mind.

* Say slowly whenever you are invaded by the thoughts about eating: sun, flower, seven, path, tee, run, yellow, apple, fish, rain, pen, water, smile, talk, life, sky.

* If above does not help to stop the thoughts about eating just turn your attention away from the invading thoughts about eating. The best way to turn your attention away from the invading thoughts about eating in your head is by doing one of your favorite occupations. Do not be ashamed of any occupation to turn your attention away from the invading thoughts in your head. ALWAYS be busy with your favorite occupation when unsupportable thoughts come to your head.

* Be careful to keep for yourself these of your believes which are found to be strange by the people.

* CONTROL what you say. Say only things which are not strange for the people. You surely already know which of your believes are found to be strange by the people.

* If you do not know yet which of your believes are found to be strange by the people, OBSERVE how people react on what you say. If you see that people are ALERTED by your believes, it means your believes are strange. From now on AVOID presenting such believes.

* Think of three different words, any words which just come to your mind at the moment and make a simple story using these 3 words. Repeat 3 times.

* Try to concentrate on an object close to you, any object. What do you feel when looking at the object? What thoughts come to your mind when looking at the object? And why? Maybe there is a reason. Look for the reason but not too long. If you don't find the reason, forget it.

* Small physical excercise (10 min)

* Small breakfast.

* Nice talk (no complaints, no problematic questions) 10 min. When nobody to talk with, phone or internet conversation oral or written.

* Walk 15 min.

* If you have invading thoughts about eating, ask yourself if it is possible to ignore them.

Yes

Great! In such a case continue ignoring them.

No

You have to learn to ignore the invading thoughts about eating.

This Guide will teach you to ignore the invading thoughts about eating.

Remember: even if you cannot stop the invading thoughts, the invading thoughts cannot stop you to live a normal life.

If you believe in things which other people consider strange, try to keep your strange believes for yourself. Everybody has to make the selection of what can be told to other people and what must be private. Believe me, many people have strange believes. Even much stranger than yours. And they are not considered to be sick. Why? Because they keep their strange believes for themselves. That is the secret.

***

Afternoon

* Say slowly whenever you are invaded by the thoughts about eating: sun, flower, seven, path, tee, run, yellow, apple, fish, rain, pen, water, smile, talk, life, sky.

* Think of three different words, any words which just come to your mind at the moment and make a simple story using these 3 words. Repeat 3 times.

* Try to concentrate on an object close to you, any object. What do you feel when looking at the object? What thoughts come to your mind when looking at the object? And why?Maybe there is a reason. Look for the reason but not too long. If you don't find the reason, forget it.

* Dinner and half an hour break (you can sleep).

* Nice talk (no complaints) 15 min. When nobody to talk with, phone or internet conversation oral or written.

* Walk 20 min.

* If you have the invading thoughts about eating, ask yourself if it is possible to ignore them.

Yes

Great! In such a case continue ignoring them.

No

You have to learn to ignore the invading thoughts.

This Guide will teach you to ignore the invading thoughts about eating.

Remember: even if you cannot stop the invading thoughts, the invading thoughts cannot stop you to live a normal life.

If you believe in things which other people consider strange, try to keep your strange believes for yourself. Everybody has to make the selection of what can be told to other people and what must be private. Believe me, many people have strange believes. Even much stranger than yours. And they are not considered to be sick. Why? Because they keep their strange believes for themselves. That is the secret.

***

Evening

- Say slowly whenever you are invaded by the thoughts about eating: sun, flower, seven, path, tee, run, yellow, apple, fish, rain, pen, water, smile, talk, life, sky.

- Think of three different words, any words which just come to your mind at the moment and make a simple story using these 3 words. Repeat 3 times.

- Try to concentrate on an object close to you, any object. What do you feel when looking at the object? What thoughts come to your mind when looking at the object? And why? Maybe there is a reason. Look for the reason but not too long. If you don't find the reason, forget it.
- Small supper.
- Nice talk (no complaints) 10 min. When nobody to talk with, phone or internet conversation oral or written.
- Walk 10 min.
- If you have the invading thoughts about eating, ask yourself if it is possible to ignore them.

Yes

Great! In such a case continue ignoring them.

No

You have to learn to ignore the invading thoughts.

This Guide will teach you to ignore the invading thoughts.

Remember: even if you cannot stop the invading thoughts, the invading thoughts cannot stop you to live a normal life.

If you believe in things which other people consider strange, try to keep your strange believes for yourself. Everybody has to make the selection of what can be told to other people and what must be private. Believe me, many people have strange believes. Even much stranger than yours. And they are not considered to be sick. Why? Because they keep their strange believes for themselves. That is the secret.

***

Night

Before sleep

- Take a shower (warm water) 1 min.
- Small physical excercise 3 min.

In Bed

- Repeat STOP (10 times if you have invading thoughts).
- Say slowly whenever you are invaded by the thoughts about eating: sun, flower, seven, path, tee, run, yellow, apple, fish, rain, pen, water, smile, talk, life, sky.
- Think of three different words, any words which just come to your mind at the moment and make a simple story using these 3 words. Repeat untill you fall asleep.

If you cannot fall asleep

- Say slowly whenever you are invaded by the thoughts about eating: sun, flower, seven, path, tee, run, yellow, apple, fish, rain, pen, water, smile, talk, life, sky.

If you cannot asleep

- Think of three different words, any words which just come to your mind at the moment and make a simple story using these 3 words. Repeat untill you fall asleep.

If above does not help

- Stand up and go to the toilet (when possible with as little light as possible)
- Say slowly whenever you are invaded by the thoughts about eating: sun, flower, seven, path, tee, run, yellow, apple, fish, rain, pen, water, smile, talk, life, sky.
- Think of three different words, any words which just come to your mind at the moment and make a simple story using these 3 words. Repeat untill you fall asleep.

If above does not help

- Say STOP untill you fall asleep

If above does not help

- Go to the kitchen and have a very small snack.
- Back to the bed think of three different words, any words which just come to your mind at the moment and make a simple story using these 3 words. Repeat untill you fall asleep.
- If above does not help think of three different words, any words which just come to your mind at the moment and make a simple story using these 3 words. Repeat untill you fall asleep.
- Say slowly whenever you are invaded by the thoughts about eating: sun, flower, seven, path, tee, run, yellow, apple, fish, rain, pen, water, smile, talk, life, sky. Repeat untill you fall asleep.

***

Day 5

Morning

* Say STOP whenever thoughts about eating come to your mind.

* Say slowly whenever you are invaded by the thoughts about eating: sun, flower, seven, path, tee, run, yellow, apple, fish, rain, pen, water, smile, talk, life, sky.

* If above does not help to stop the thoughts about eating just turn your attention away from the invading thoughts about eating. The best way to turn your attention away from the invading thoughts about eating in your head is by doing one of your favorite occupations. Do not be ashamed of any occupation to turn your attention away from the invading thoughts in your head. ALWAYS be busy with your favorite occupation when unsupportable thoughts come to your head.

* Be careful to keep for yourself these of your believes which are found to be strange by the people.

* CONTROL what you say. Say only things which are not strange for the people. You surely already know which of your believes are found to be strange by the people.

* If you do not know yet which of your believes are found to be strange by the people, OBSERVE how people react on what you say. If you see that people are ALERTED by your believes, it means your believes are strange. From now on AVOID presenting such believes.

* Think of three different words, any words which just come to your mind at the moment and make a simple story using these 3 words. Repeat 3 times.

* Try to concentrate on an object close to you, any object. What do you feel when looking at the object? What thoughts come to your mind when looking at the object? And why? Maybe there is a reason. Look for the reason but not too long. If you don't find the reason, forget it.

* Small physical excercise (10 min)

* Small breakfast.

* Nice talk (no complaints, no problematic questions) 10 min. When nobody to talk with, phone or internet conversation oral or written.

* Walk 15 min.

* If you have invading thoughts about eating, ask yourself if it is possible to ignore them.

Yes

Great! In such a case continue ignoring them.

No

You have to learn to ignore the invading thoughts about eating.

This Guide will teach you to ignore the invading thoughts about eating.

Remember: even if you cannot stop the invading thoughts, the invading thoughts cannot stop you to live a normal life.

If you believe in things which other people consider strange, try to keep your strange believes for yourself. Everybody has to make the selection of what can be told to other people and what must be private. Believe me, many people have strange believes. Even much stranger than yours. And they are not considered to be sick. Why? Because they keep their strange believes for themselves. That is the secret.

***

Afternoon

* Say slowly whenever you are invaded by the thoughts about eating: sun, flower, seven, path, tee, run, yellow, apple, fish, rain, pen, water, smile, talk, life, sky.

* Think of three different words, any words which just come to your mind at the moment and make a simple story using these 3 words. Repeat 3 times.

* Try to concentrate on an object close to you, any object. What do you feel when looking at the object? What thoughts come to your mind when looking at the

object? And why? Maybe there is a reason. Look for the reason but not too long. If you don't find the reason, forget it.

* Dinner and half an hour break (you can sleep).

* Nice talk (no complaints) 15 min. When nobody to talk with, phone or internet conversation oral or written.

* Walk 20 min.

* If you have the invading thoughts about eating, ask yourself if it is possible to ignore them.

Yes

Great! In such a case continue ignoring them.

No

You have to learn to ignore the invading thoughts.

This Guide will teach you to ignore the invading thoughts about eating.

Remember: even if you cannot stop the invading thoughts, the invading thoughts cannot stop you to live a normal life.

If you believe in things which other people consider strange, try to keep your strange believes for yourself. Everybody has to make the selection of what can be

told to other people and what must be private. Believe me, many people have strange believes. Even much stranger than yours. And they are not considered to be sick. Why? Because they keep their strange believes for themselves. That is the secret.

***

Evening

- Say slowly whenever you are invaded by the thoughts about eating: sun, flower, seven, path, tee, run, yellow, apple, fish, rain, pen, water, smile, talk, life, sky.

- Think of three different words, any words which just come to your mind at the moment and make a simple story using these 3 words. Repeat 3 times.
  - Try to concentrate on an object close to you, any object. What do you feel when looking at the object? What thoughts come to your mind when looking at the object? And why? Maybe there is a reason. Look for the reason but not too long. If you don't find the reason, forget it.
  - Small supper.
  - Nice talk (no complaints) 10 min. When nobody to talk with, phone or internet conversation oral or written.

- Walk 10 min.
- If you have the invading thoughts about eating, ask yourself if it is possible to ignore them.

Yes

Great! In such a case continue ignoring them.

No

You have to learn to ignore the invading thoughts.

This Guide will teach you to ignore the invading thoughts.

Remember: even if you cannot stop the invading thoughts, the invading thoughts cannot stop you to live a normal life.

If you believe in things which other people consider strange, try to keep your strange believes for yourself. Everybody has to make the selection of what can be told to other people and what must be private. Believe me, many people have strange believes. Even much stranger than yours. And they are not considered to be sick. Why? Because they keep their strange believes for themselves. That is the secret.

***

Night

Before sleep

- Take a shower (warm water) 1 min.
- Small physical excercise 3 min.

In Bed

- Repeat STOP (10 times if you have invading thoughts).
- Say slowly whenever you are invaded by the thoughts about eating: sun, flower, seven, path, tee, run, yellow, apple, fish, rain, pen, water, smile, talk, life, sky.
- Think of three different words, any words which just come to your mind at the moment and make a simple story using these 3 words. Repeat untill you fall asleep.

If you cannot fall asleep

- Say slowly whenever you are invaded by the thoughts about eating: sun, flower, seven, path, tee, run, yellow, apple, fish, rain, pen, water, smile, talk, life, sky.

If you cannot asleep

- Think of three different words, any words which just come to your mind at the moment and make a simple story using these 3 words. Repeat untill you fall asleep.

If above does not help

- Stand up and go to the toilet (when possible with as little light as possible)
- Say slowly whenever you are invaded by the thoughts about eating: sun, flower, seven, path, tee, run, yellow, apple, fish, rain, pen, water, smile, talk, life, sky.
- Think of three different words, any words which just come to your mind at the moment and make a simple story using these 3 words. Repeat untill you fall asleep.

If above does not help

- Say STOP untill you fall asleep

If above does not help

- Go to the kitchen and have a very small snack.
- Back to the bed think of three different words, any words which just come to your mind at the moment and make a simple story using these 3 words. Repeat untill you fall asleep.
- If above does not help think of three different words, any words which just come to your mind at the moment and make a simple story using these 3 words. Repeat untill you fall asleep.

- Say slowly whenever you are invaded by the thoughts about eating: sun, flower, seven, path, tee, run, yellow, apple, fish, rain, pen, water, smile, talk, life, sky. Repeat untill you fall asleep.

***

Day 6

Morning

* Say STOP whenever thoughts about eating come to your mind.

* Say slowly whenever you are invaded by the thoughts about eating: sun, flower, seven, path, tee, run, yellow, apple, fish, rain, pen, water, smile, talk, life, sky.

* If above does not help to stop the thoughts about eating just turn your attention away from the invading thoughts about eating. The best way to turn your attention away from the invading thoughts about eating in your head is by doing one of your favorite occupations. Do not be ashamed of any occupation to turn your attention away from the invading thoughts in your head. ALWAYS be busy with your favorite occupation when unsupportable thoughts come to your head.

* Be careful to keep for yourself these of your believes which are found to be strange by the people.

* CONTROL what you say. Say only things which are not strange for the people. You surely already know which of your believes are found to be strange by the people.

* If you do not know yet which of your believes are found to be strange by the people, OBSERVE how people react on what you say. If you see that people are ALERTED by your believes, it means your believes are strange. From now on AVOID presenting such believes.

* Think of three different words, any words which just come to your mind at the moment and make a simple story using these 3 words. Repeat 3 times.

* Try to concentrate on an object close to you, any object. What do you feel when looking at the object? What thoughts come to your mind when looking at the object? And why?Maybe there is a reason. Look for the reason but not too long. If you don't find the reason, forget it.

* Small physical excercise (10 min)

* Small breakfast.

* Nice talk (no complaints, no problematic questions) 10 min. When nobody to talk with, phone or internet conversation oral or written.

* Walk 15 min.

* If you have invading thoughts about eating, ask yourself if it is possible to ignore them.

Yes

Great! In such a case continue ignoring them.

No

You have to learn to ignore the invading thoughts about eating.

This Guide will teach you to ignore the invading thoughts about eating.

Remember: even if you cannot stop the invading thoughts, the invading thoughts cannot stop you to live a normal life.

If you believe in things which other people consider strange, try to keep your strange believes for yourself. Everybody has to make the selection of what can be told to other people and what must be private. Believe me, many people have strange believes. Even much stranger than yours. And they are not considered to be

sick. Why? Because they keep their strange believes for themselves. That is the secret.

***

Afternoon

* Say slowly whenever you are invaded by the thoughts about eating: sun, flower, seven, path, tee, run, yellow, apple, fish, rain, pen, water, smile, talk, life, sky.

* Think of three different words, any words which just come to your mind at the moment and make a simple story using these 3 words. Repeat 3 times.

* Try to concentrate on an object close to you, any object. What do you feel when looking at the object? What thoughts come to your mind when looking at the object? And why?Maybe there is a reason. Look for the reason but not too long. If you don't find the reason, forget it.

* Dinner and half an hour break (you can sleep).

* Nice talk (no complaints) 15 min. When nobody to talk with, phone or internet conversation oral or written.

* Walk 20 min.

* If you have the invading thoughts about eating, ask yourself if it is possible to ignore them.

Yes

Great! In such a case continue ignoring them.

No

You have to learn to ignore the invading thoughts.

This Guide will teach you to ignore the invading thoughts about eating.

Remember: even if you cannot stop the invading thoughts, the invading thoughts cannot stop you to live a normal life.

If you believe in things which other people consider strange, try to keep your strange believes for yourself. Everybody has to make the selection of what can be told to other people and what must be private. Believe me, many people have strange believes. Even much stranger than yours. And they are not considered to be sick. Why? Because they keep their strange believes for themselves. That is the secret.

***

Evening

- Say slowly whenever you are invaded by the thoughts about eating: sun, flower, seven, path, tee, run, yellow, apple, fish, rain, pen, water, smile, talk, life, sky.

- Think of three different words, any words which just come to your mind at the moment and make a simple story using these 3 words. Repeat 3 times.
  - Try to concentrate on an object close to you, any object. What do you feel when looking at the object? What thoughts come to your mind when looking at the object? And why? Maybe there is a reason. Look for the reason but not too long. If you don't find the reason, forget it.
  - Small supper.
  - Nice talk (no complaints) 10 min. When nobody to talk with, phone or internet conversation oral or written.
  - Walk 10 min.
  - If you have the invading thoughts about eating, ask yourself if it is possible to ignore them.

Yes

Great! In such a case continue ignoring them.

No

You have to learn to ignore the invading thoughts.

This Guide will teach you to ignore the invading thoughts.

Remember: even if you cannot stop the invading thoughts, the invading thoughts cannot stop you to live a normal life.

If you believe in things which other people consider strange, try to keep your strange believes for yourself. Everybody has to make the selection of what can be told to other people and what must be private. Believe me, many people have strange believes. Even much stranger than yours. And they are not considered to be sick. Why? Because they keep their strange believes for themselves. That is the secret.

***

Night

Before sleep

- Take a shower (warm water) 1 min.
- Small physical excercise 3 min.

In Bed

- Repeat STOP (10 times if you have invading thoughts).

- Say slowly whenever you are invaded by the thoughts about eating: sun, flower, seven, path, tee, run, yellow, apple, fish, rain, pen, water, smile, talk, life, sky.
- Think of three different words, any words which just come to your mind at the moment and make a simple story using these 3 words. Repeat untill you fall asleep.

If you cannot fall asleep

- Say slowly whenever you are invaded by the thoughts about eating: sun, flower, seven, path, tee, run, yellow, apple, fish, rain, pen, water, smile, talk, life, sky.

If you cannot asleep

- Think of three different words, any words which just come to your mind at the moment and make a simple story using these 3 words. Repeat untill you fall asleep.

If above does not help

- Stand up and go to the toilet (when possible with as little light as possible)
- Say slowly whenever you are invaded by the thoughts about eating: sun, flower, seven, path,

tee, run, yellow, apple, fish, rain, pen, water, smile, talk, life, sky.
- Think of three different words, any words which just come to your mind at the moment and make a simple story using these 3 words. Repeat untill you fall asleep.

If above does not help
- Say STOP untill you fall asleep

If above does not help
- Go to the kitchen and have a very small snack.
- Back to the bed think of three different words, any words which just come to your mind at the moment and make a simple story using these 3 words. Repeat untill you fall asleep.
- If above does not help think of three different words, any words which just come to your mind at the moment and make a simple story using these 3 words. Repeat untill you fall asleep.
- Say slowly whenever you are invaded by the thoughts about eating: sun, flower, seven, path, tee, run, yellow, apple, fish, rain, pen, water, smile, talk, life, sky. Repeat untill you fall asleep.

***

Day 7

Morning

* Say STOP whenever thoughts about eating come to your mind.

* Say slowly whenever you are invaded by the thoughts about eating: sun, flower, seven, path, tee, run, yellow, apple, fish, rain, pen, water, smile, talk, life, sky.

* If above does not help to stop the thoughts about eating just turn your attention away from the invading thoughts about eating. The best way to turn your attention away from the invading thoughts about eating in your head is by doing one of your favorite occupations. Do not be ashamed of any occupation to turn your attention away from the invading thoughts in your head. ALWAYS be busy with your favorite occupation when unsupportable thoughts come to your head.

* Be careful to keep for yourself these of your believes which are found to be strange by the people.

* CONTROL what you say. Say only things which are not strange for the people. You surely already know which of your believes are found to be strange by the people.

* If you do not know yet which of your believes are found to be strange by the people, OBSERVE how

people react on what you say. If you see that people are ALERTED by your believes, it means your believes are strange. From now on AVOID presenting such believes.

* Think of three different words, any words which just come to your mind at the moment and make a simple story using these 3 words. Repeat 3 times.

* Try to concentrate on an object close to you, any object. What do you feel when looking at the object? What thoughts come to your mind when looking at the object? And why? Maybe there is a reason. Look for the reason but not too long. If you don't find the reason, forget it.

* Small physical excercise (10 min)

* Small breakfast.

* Nice talk (no complaints, no problematic questions) 10 min. When nobody to talk with, phone or internet conversation oral or written.

* Walk 15 min.

* If you have invading thoughts about eating, ask yourself if it is possible to ignore them.

Yes

Great! In such a case continue ignoring them.

No

You have to learn to ignore the invading thoughts about eating.

This Guide will teach you to ignore the invading thoughts about eating.

Remember: even if you cannot stop the invading thoughts, the invading thoughts cannot stop you to live a normal life.

If you believe in things which other people consider strange, try to keep your strange believes for yourself. Everybody has to make the selection of what can be told to other people and what must be private. Believe me, many people have strange believes. Even much stranger than yours. And they are not considered to be sick. Why? Because they keep their strange believes for themselves. That is the secret.

***

Afternoon

* Say slowly whenever you are invaded by the thoughts about eating: sun, flower, seven, path, tee, run, yellow, apple, fish, rain, pen, water, smile, talk, life, sky.

* Think of three different words, any words which just come to your mind at the moment and make a simple story using these 3 words. Repeat 3 times.

* Try to concentrate on an object close to you, any object. What do you feel when looking at the object? What thoughts come to your mind when looking at the object? And why? Maybe there is a reason. Look for the reason but not too long. If you don't find the reason, forget it.

* Dinner and half an hour break (you can sleep).

* Nice talk (no complaints) 15 min. When nobody to talk with, phone or internet conversation oral or written.

* Walk 20 min.

* If you have the invading thoughts about eating, ask yourself if it is possible to ignore them.

Yes

Great! In such a case continue ignoring them.

No

You have to learn to ignore the invading thoughts.

This Guide will teach you to ignore the invading thoughts about eating.

Remember: even if you cannot stop the invading thoughts, the invading thoughts cannot stop you to live a normal life.

If you believe in things which other people consider strange, try to keep your strange believes for yourself. Everybody has to make the selection of what can be told to other people and what must be private. Believe me, many people have strange believes. Even much stranger than yours. And they are not considered to be sick. Why? Because they keep their strange believes for themselves. That is the secret.

***

Evening

- Say slowly whenever you are invaded by the thoughts about eating: sun, flower, seven, path, tee, run, yellow, apple, fish, rain, pen, water, smile, talk, life, sky.

- Think of three different words, any words which just come to your mind at the moment and make a simple story using these 3 words. Repeat 3 times.
    - Try to concentrate on an object close to you, any object. What do you feel when looking at the object? What thoughts come to your mind when

looking at the object? And why? Maybe there is a reason. Look for the reason but not too long. If you don't find the reason, forget it.
- Small supper.
- Nice talk (no complaints) 10 min. When nobody to talk with, phone or internet conversation oral or written.
- Walk 10 min.
- If you have the invading thoughts about eating, ask yourself if it is possible to ignore them.

Yes

Great! In such a case continue ignoring them.

No

You have to learn to ignore the invading thoughts.

This Guide will teach you to ignore the invading thoughts.

Remember: even if you cannot stop the invading thoughts, the invading thoughts cannot stop you to live a normal life.

If you believe in things which other people consider strange, try to keep your strange believes for yourself. Everybody has to make the selection of what can be told to other people and what must be private. Believe

me, many people have strange believes. Even much stranger than yours. And they are not considered to be sick. Why? Because they keep their strange believes for themselves. That is the secret.

***

Night

Before sleep

- Take a shower (warm water) 1 min.
- Small physical excercise 3 min.

In Bed

- Repeat STOP (10 times if you have invading thoughts).
- Say slowly whenever you are invaded by the thoughts about eating: sun, flower, seven, path, tee, run, yellow, apple, fish, rain, pen, water, smile, talk, life, sky.
- Think of three different words, any words which just come to your mind at the moment and make a simple story using these 3 words. Repeat untill you fall asleep.

If you cannot fall asleep

- Say slowly whenever you are invaded by the thoughts about eating: sun, flower, seven, path,

tee, run, yellow, apple, fish, rain, pen, water, smile, talk, life, sky.

If you cannot asleep

- Think of three different words, any words which just come to your mind at the moment and make a simple story using these 3 words. Repeat untill you fall asleep.

If above does not help

- Stand up and go to the toilet (when possible with as little light as possible)
- Say slowly whenever you are invaded by the thoughts about eating: sun, flower, seven, path, tee, run, yellow, apple, fish, rain, pen, water, smile, talk, life, sky.
- Think of three different words, any words which just come to your mind at the moment and make a simple story using these 3 words. Repeat untill you fall asleep.

If above does not help

- Say STOP untill you fall asleep

If above does not help

- Go to the kitchen and have a very small snack.

- Back to the bed think of three different words, any words which just come to your mind at the moment and make a simple story using these 3 words. Repeat untill you fall asleep.
- If above does not help think of three different words, any words which just come to your mind at the moment and make a simple story using these 3 words. Repeat untill you fall asleep.
- Say slowly whenever you are invaded by the thoughts about eating: sun, flower, seven, path, tee, run, yellow, apple, fish, rain, pen, water, smile, talk, life, sky. Repeat untill you fall asleep.

***

Week Eight

Day 1

Morning

* Say STOP whenever thoughts about eating come to your mind.

* Say slowly whenever you are invaded by the thoughts about eating: sun, flower, seven, path, tee, run, yellow, apple, fish, rain, pen, water, smile, talk, life, sky.

* If above does not help to stop the thoughts about eating just turn your attention away from the invading thoughts about eating. The best way to turn your attention away from the invading thoughts about eating in your head is by doing one of your favorite occupations. Do not be ashamed of any occupation to turn your attention away from the invading thoughts in your head. ALWAYS be busy with your favorite occupation when unsupportable thoughts come to your head.

* Be careful to keep for yourself these of your believes which are found to be strange by the people.

* CONTROL what you say. Say only things which are not strange for the people. You surely already know which of your believes are found to be strange by the people.

* If you do not know yet which of your believes are found to be strange by the people, OBSERVE how people react on what you say. If you see that people are ALERTED by your believes, it means your believes are strange. From now on AVOID presenting such believes.

* Think of three different words, any words which just come to your mind at the moment and make a simple story using these 3 words. Repeat 3 times.

* Try to concentrate on an object close to you, any object. What do you feel when looking at the object? What thoughts come to your mind when looking at the

object? And why? Maybe there is a reason. Look for the reason but not too long. If you don't find the reason, forget it.

* Small physical excercise (10 min)

* Small breakfast.

* Nice talk (no complaints, no problematic questions) 10 min. When nobody to talk with, phone or internet conversation oral or written.

* Walk 15 min.

* If you have invading thoughts about eating, ask yourself if it is possible to ignore them.

Yes

Great! In such a case continue ignoring them.

No

You have to learn to ignore the invading thoughts about eating.

This Guide will teach you to ignore the invading thoughts about eating.

Remember: even if you cannot stop the invading thoughts, the invading thoughts cannot stop you to live a normal life.

If you believe in things which other people consider strange, try to keep your strange believes for yourself. Everybody has to make the selection of what can be told to other people and what must be private. Believe me, many people have strange believes. Even much stranger than yours. And they are not considered to be sick. Why? Because they keep their strange believes for themselves. That is the secret.

***

Afternoon

* Say slowly whenever you are invaded by the thoughts about eating: sun, flower, seven, path, tee, run, yellow, apple, fish, rain, pen, water, smile, talk, life, sky.

* Think of three different words, any words which just come to your mind at the moment and make a simple story using these 3 words. Repeat 3 times.

* Try to concentrate on an object close to you, any object. What do you feel when looking at the object? What thoughts come to your mind when looking at the object? And why? Maybe there is a reason. Look for the reason but not too long. If you don't find the reason, forget it.

* Dinner and half an hour break (you can sleep).

* Nice talk (no complaints) 15 min. When nobody to talk with, phone or internet conversation oral or written.

* Walk 20 min.

* If you have the invading thoughts about eating, ask yourself if it is possible to ignore them.

Yes

Great! In such a case continue ignoring them.

No

You have to learn to ignore the invading thoughts.

This Guide will teach you to ignore the invading thoughts about eating.

Remember: even if you cannot stop the invading thoughts, the invading thoughts cannot stop you to live a normal life.

If you believe in things which other people consider strange, try to keep your strange believes for yourself. Everybody has to make the selection of what can be told to other people and what must be private. Believe me, many people have strange believes. Even much stranger than yours. And they are not considered to be

sick. Why? Because they keep their strange believes for themselves. That is the secret.

***

Evening

- Say slowly whenever you are invaded by the thoughts about eating: sun, flower, seven, path, tee, run, yellow, apple, fish, rain, pen, water, smile, talk, life, sky.

- Think of three different words, any words which just come to your mind at the moment and make a simple story using these 3 words. Repeat 3 times.
  - Try to concentrate on an object close to you, any object. What do you feel when looking at the object? What thoughts come to your mind when looking at the object? And why? Maybe there is a reason. Look for the reason but not too long. If you don't find the reason, forget it.
  - Small supper.
  - Nice talk (no complaints) 10 min. When nobody to talk with, phone or internet conversation oral or written.
  - Walk 10 min.
  - If you have the invading thoughts about eating, ask yourself if it is possible to ignore them.

Yes

Great! In such a case continue ignoring them.

No

You have to learn to ignore the invading thoughts.

This Guide will teach you to ignore the invading thoughts.

Remember: even if you cannot stop the invading thoughts, the invading thoughts cannot stop you to live a normal life.

If you believe in things which other people consider strange, try to keep your strange believes for yourself. Everybody has to make the selection of what can be told to other people and what must be private. Believe me, many people have strange believes. Even much stranger than yours. And they are not considered to be sick. Why? Because they keep their strange believes for themselves. That is the secret.

***

Night

Before sleep

- Take a shower (warm water) 1 min.
- Small physical excercise 3 min.

In Bed

- Repeat STOP (10 times if you have invading thoughts).
- Say slowly whenever you are invaded by the thoughts about eating: sun, flower, seven, path, tee, run, yellow, apple, fish, rain, pen, water, smile, talk, life, sky.
- Think of three different words, any words which just come to your mind at the moment and make a simple story using these 3 words. Repeat untill you fall asleep.

If you cannot fall asleep

- Say slowly whenever you are invaded by the thoughts about eating: sun, flower, seven, path, tee, run, yellow, apple, fish, rain, pen, water, smile, talk, life, sky.

If you cannot asleep

- Think of three different words, any words which just come to your mind at the moment and make a simple story using these 3 words. Repeat untill you fall asleep.

If above does not help

- Stand up and go to the toilet (when possible with as little light as possible)

- Say slowly whenever you are invaded by the thoughts about eating: sun, flower, seven, path, tee, run, yellow, apple, fish, rain, pen, water, smile, talk, life, sky.
- Think of three different words, any words which just come to your mind at the moment and make a simple story using these 3 words. Repeat untill you fall asleep.

If above does not help

- Say STOP untill you fall asleep

If above does not help

- Go to the kitchen and have a very small snack.
- Back to the bed think of three different words, any words which just come to your mind at the moment and make a simple story using these 3 words. Repeat untill you fall asleep.
- If above does not help think of three different words, any words which just come to your mind at the moment and make a simple story using these 3 words. Repeat untill you fall asleep.
- Say slowly whenever you are invaded by the thoughts about eating: sun, flower, seven, path, tee, run, yellow, apple, fish, rain, pen, water, smile, talk, life, sky. Repeat untill you fall asleep.

***

Day 2

Morning

* Say STOP whenever thoughts about eating come to your mind.

* Say slowly whenever you are invaded by the thoughts about eating: sun, flower, seven, path, tee, run, yellow, apple, fish, rain, pen, water, smile, talk, life, sky.

* If above does not help to stop the thoughts about eating just turn your attention away from the invading thoughts about eating. The best way to turn your attention away from the invading thoughts about eating in your head is by doing one of your favorite occupations. Do not be ashamed of any occupation to turn your attention away from the invading thoughts in your head. ALWAYS be busy with your favorite occupation when unsupportable thoughts come to your head.

* Be careful to keep for yourself these of your believes which are found to be strange by the people.

* CONTROL what you say. Say only things which are not strange for the people. You surely already know which of your believes are found to be strange by the people.

* If you do not know yet which of your believes are found to be strange by the people, OBSERVE how people react on what you say. If you see that people are ALERTED by your believes, it means your believes are strange. From now on AVOID presenting such believes.

* Think of three different words, any words which just come to your mind at the moment and make a simple story using these 3 words. Repeat 3 times.

* Try to concentrate on an object close to you, any object. What do you feel when looking at the object? What thoughts come to your mind when looking at the object? And why? Maybe there is a reason. Look for the reason but not too long. If you don't find the reason, forget it.

* Small physical excercise (10 min)

* Small breakfast.

* Nice talk (no complaints, no problematic questions) 10 min. When nobody to talk with, phone or internet conversation oral or written.

* Walk 15 min.

* If you have invading thoughts about eating, ask yourself if it is possible to ignore them.

Yes

Great! In such a case continue ignoring them.

No

You have to learn to ignore the invading thoughts about eating.

This Guide will teach you to ignore the invading thoughts about eating.

Remember: even if you cannot stop the invading thoughts, the invading thoughts cannot stop you to live a normal life.

If you believe in things which other people consider strange, try to keep your strange believes for yourself. Everybody has to make the selection of what can be told to other people and what must be private. Believe me, many people have strange believes. Even much stranger than yours. And they are not considered to be sick. Why? Because they keep their strange believes for themselves. That is the secret.

***

Afternoon

* Say slowly whenever you are invaded by the thoughts about eating: sun, flower, seven, path, tee, run, yellow, apple, fish, rain, pen, water, smile, talk, life, sky.

* Think of three different words, any words which just come to your mind at the moment and make a simple story using these 3 words. Repeat 3 times.

* Try to concentrate on an object close to you, any object. What do you feel when looking at the object? What thoughts come to your mind when looking at the object? And why? Maybe there is a reason. Look for the reason but not too long. If you don't find the reason, forget it.

* Dinner and half an hour break (you can sleep).

* Nice talk (no complaints) 15 min. When nobody to talk with, phone or internet conversation oral or written.

* Walk 20 min.

* If you have the invading thoughts about eating, ask yourself if it is possible to ignore them.

Yes

Great! In such a case continue ignoring them.

No

You have to learn to ignore the invading thoughts.

This Guide will teach you to ignore the invading thoughts about eating.

Remember: even if you cannot stop the invading thoughts, the invading thoughts cannot stop you to live a normal life.

If you believe in things which other people consider strange, try to keep your strange believes for yourself. Everybody has to make the selection of what can be told to other people and what must be private. Believe me, many people have strange believes. Even much stranger than yours. And they are not considered to be sick. Why? Because they keep their strange believes for themselves. That is the secret.

***

Evening

- Say slowly whenever you are invaded by the thoughts about eating: sun, flower, seven, path, tee, run, yellow, apple, fish, rain, pen, water, smile, talk, life, sky.

- Think of three different words, any words which just come to your mind at the moment and make a simple story using these 3 words. Repeat 3 times.

- Try to concentrate on an object close to you, any object. What do you feel when looking at the object? What thoughts come to your mind when looking at the object? And why? Maybe there is a reason. Look for the reason but not too long. If you don't find the reason, forget it.
- Small supper.
- Nice talk (no complaints) 10 min. When nobody to talk with, phone or internet conversation oral or written.
- Walk 10 min.
- If you have the invading thoughts about eating, ask yourself if it is possible to ignore them.

Yes

Great! In such a case continue ignoring them.

No

You have to learn to ignore the invading thoughts.

This Guide will teach you to ignore the invading thoughts.

Remember: even if you cannot stop the invading thoughts, the invading thoughts cannot stop you to live a normal life.

If you believe in things which other people consider strange, try to keep your strange believes for yourself. Everybody has to make the selection of what can be told to other people and what must be private. Believe me, many people have strange believes. Even much stranger than yours. And they are not considered to be sick. Why? Because they keep their strange believes for themselves. That is the secret.

***

Night

Before sleep

- Take a shower (warm water) 1 min.
- Small physical excercise 3 min.

In Bed

- Repeat STOP (10 times if you have invading thoughts).
- Say slowly whenever you are invaded by the thoughts about eating: sun, flower, seven, path, tee, run, yellow, apple, fish, rain, pen, water, smile, talk, life, sky.
- Think of three different words, any words which just come to your mind at the moment and make a simple story using these 3 words. Repeat untill you fall asleep.

If you cannot fall asleep

- Say slowly whenever you are invaded by the thoughts about eating: sun, flower, seven, path, tee, run, yellow, apple, fish, rain, pen, water, smile, talk, life, sky.

If you cannot asleep

- Think of three different words, any words which just come to your mind at the moment and make a simple story using these 3 words. Repeat untill you fall asleep.

If above does not help

- Stand up and go to the toilet (when possible with as little light as possible)
- Say slowly whenever you are invaded by the thoughts about eating: sun, flower, seven, path, tee, run, yellow, apple, fish, rain, pen, water, smile, talk, life, sky.
- Think of three different words, any words which just come to your mind at the moment and make a simple story using these 3 words. Repeat untill you fall asleep.

If above does not help

- Say STOP untill you fall asleep

If above does not help

- Go to the kitchen and have a very small snack.
- Back to the bed think of three different words, any words which just come to your mind at the moment and make a simple story using these 3 words. Repeat untill you fall asleep.
- If above does not help think of three different words, any words which just come to your mind at the moment and make a simple story using these 3 words. Repeat untill you fall asleep.
- Say slowly whenever you are invaded by the thoughts about eating: sun, flower, seven, path, tee, run, yellow, apple, fish, rain, pen, water, smile, talk, life, sky. Repeat untill you fall asleep.

***

Day 3

Morning

* Say STOP whenever thoughts about eating come to your mind.

* Say slowly whenever you are invaded by the thoughts about eating: sun, flower, seven, path, tee, run, yellow, apple, fish, rain, pen, water, smile, talk, life, sky.

* If above does not help to stop the thoughts about eating just turn your attention away from the invading thoughts about eating. The best way to turn your attention away from the invading thoughts about eating in your head is by doing one of your favorite occupations. Do not be ashamed of any occupation to turn your attention away from the invading thoughts in your head. ALWAYS be busy with your favorite occupation when unsupportable thoughts come to your head.

* Be careful to keep for yourself these of your believes which are found to be strange by the people.

* CONTROL what you say. Say only things which are not strange for the people. You surely already know which of your believes are found to be strange by the people.

* If you do not know yet which of your believes are found to be strange by the people, OBSERVE how people react on what you say. If you see that people are ALERTED by your believes, it means your believes are strange. From now on AVOID presenting such believes.

* Think of three different words, any words which just come to your mind at the moment and make a simple story using these 3 words. Repeat 3 times.

* Try to concentrate on an object close to you, any object. What do you feel when looking at the object? What thoughts come to your mind when looking at the object? And why? Maybe there is a reason. Look for the reason but not too long. If you don't find the reason, forget it.

* Small physical excercise (10 min)

* Small breakfast.

* Nice talk (no complaints, no problematic questions) 10 min. When nobody to talk with, phone or internet conversation oral or written.

* Walk 15 min.

* If you have invading thoughts about eating, ask yourself if it is possible to ignore them.

Yes

Great! In such a case continue ignoring them.

No

You have to learn to ignore the invading thoughts about eating.

This Guide will teach you to ignore the invading thoughts about eating.

Remember: even if you cannot stop the invading thoughts, the invading thoughts cannot stop you to live a normal life.

If you believe in things which other people consider strange, try to keep your strange believes for yourself. Everybody has to make the selection of what can be told to other people and what must be private. Believe me, many people have strange believes. Even much stranger than yours. And they are not considered to be sick. Why? Because they keep their strange believes for themselves. That is the secret.

***

Afternoon

* Say slowly whenever you are invaded by the thoughts about eating: sun, flower, seven, path, tee, run, yellow, apple, fish, rain, pen, water, smile, talk, life, sky.

* Think of three different words, any words which just come to your mind at the moment and make a simple story using these 3 words. Repeat 3 times.

* Try to concentrate on an object close to you, any object. What do you feel when looking at the object? What thoughts come to your mind when looking at the

object? And why? Maybe there is a reason. Look for the reason but not too long. If you don't find the reason, forget it.

* Dinner and half an hour break (you can sleep).

* Nice talk (no complaints) 15 min. When nobody to talk with, phone or internet conversation oral or written.

* Walk 20 min.

* If you have the invading thoughts about eating, ask yourself if it is possible to ignore them.

Yes

Great! In such a case continue ignoring them.

No

You have to learn to ignore the invading thoughts.

This Guide will teach you to ignore the invading thoughts about eating.

Remember: even if you cannot stop the invading thoughts, the invading thoughts cannot stop you to live a normal life.

If you believe in things which other people consider strange, try to keep your strange believes for yourself. Everybody has to make the selection of what can be

told to other people and what must be private. Believe me, many people have strange believes. Even much stranger than yours. And they are not considered to be sick. Why? Because they keep their strange believes for themselves. That is the secret.

***

Evening

- Say slowly whenever you are invaded by the thoughts about eating: sun, flower, seven, path, tee, run, yellow, apple, fish, rain, pen, water, smile, talk, life, sky.

- Think of three different words, any words which just come to your mind at the moment and make a simple story using these 3 words. Repeat 3 times.
    - Try to concentrate on an object close to you, any object. What do you feel when looking at the object? What thoughts come to your mind when looking at the object? And why? Maybe there is a reason. Look for the reason but not too long. If you don't find the reason, forget it.
    - Small supper.
    - Nice talk (no complaints) 10 min. When nobody to talk with, phone or internet conversation oral or written.

- Walk 10 min.
- If you have the invading thoughts about eating, ask yourself if it is possible to ignore them.

Yes

Great! In such a case continue ignoring them.

No

You have to learn to ignore the invading thoughts.

This Guide will teach you to ignore the invading thoughts.

Remember: even if you cannot stop the invading thoughts, the invading thoughts cannot stop you to live a normal life.

If you believe in things which other people consider strange, try to keep your strange believes for yourself. Everybody has to make the selection of what can be told to other people and what must be private. Believe me, many people have strange believes. Even much stranger than yours. And they are not considered to be sick. Why? Because they keep their strange believes for themselves. That is the secret.

***

Night

Before sleep

- Take a shower (warm water) 1 min.
- Small physical excercise 3 min.

In Bed

- Repeat STOP (10 times if you have invading thoughts).
- Say slowly whenever you are invaded by the thoughts about eating: sun, flower, seven, path, tee, run, yellow, apple, fish, rain, pen, water, smile, talk, life, sky.
- Think of three different words, any words which just come to your mind at the moment and make a simple story using these 3 words. Repeat untill you fall asleep.

If you cannot fall asleep

- Say slowly whenever you are invaded by the thoughts about eating: sun, flower, seven, path, tee, run, yellow, apple, fish, rain, pen, water, smile, talk, life, sky.

If you cannot asleep

- Think of three different words, any words which just come to your mind at the moment and make a simple story using these 3 words. Repeat untill you fall asleep.

If above does not help

- Stand up and go to the toilet (when possible with as little light as possible)
- Say slowly whenever you are invaded by the thoughts about eating: sun, flower, seven, path, tee, run, yellow, apple, fish, rain, pen, water, smile, talk, life, sky.
- Think of three different words, any words which just come to your mind at the moment and make a simple story using these 3 words. Repeat untill you fall asleep.

If above does not help

- Say STOP untill you fall asleep

If above does not help

- Go to the kitchen and have a very small snack.
- Back to the bed think of three different words, any words which just come to your mind at the moment and make a simple story using these 3 words. Repeat untill you fall asleep.
- If above does not help think of three different words, any words which just come to your mind at the moment and make a simple story using these 3 words. Repeat untill you fall asleep.

- Say slowly whenever you are invaded by the thoughts about eating: sun, flower, seven, path, tee, run, yellow, apple, fish, rain, pen, water, smile, talk, life, sky. Repeat untill you fall asleep.

***

Day 4

Morning

* Say STOP whenever thoughts about eating come to your mind.

* Say slowly whenever you are invaded by the thoughts about eating: sun, flower, seven, path, tee, run, yellow, apple, fish, rain, pen, water, smile, talk, life, sky.

* If above does not help to stop the thoughts about eating just turn your attention away from the invading thoughts about eating. The best way to turn your attention away from the invading thoughts about eating in your head is by doing one of your favorite occupations. Do not be ashamed of any occupation to turn your attention away from the invading thoughts in your head. ALWAYS be busy with your favorite occupation when unsupportable thoughts come to your head.

* Be careful to keep for yourself these of your believes which are found to be strange by the people.

* CONTROL what you say. Say only things which are not strange for the people. You surely already know which of your believes are found to be strange by the people.

* If you do not know yet which of your believes are found to be strange by the people, OBSERVE how people react on what you say. If you see that people are ALERTED by your believes, it means your believes are strange. From now on AVOID presenting such believes.

* Think of three different words, any words which just come to your mind at the moment and make a simple story using these 3 words. Repeat 3 times.

* Try to concentrate on an object close to you, any object. What do you feel when looking at the object? What thoughts come to your mind when looking at the object? And why? Maybe there is a reason. Look for the reason but not too long. If you don't find the reason, forget it.

* Small physical excercise (10 min)

* Small breakfast.

* Nice talk (no complaints, no problematic questions) 10 min. When nobody to talk with, phone or internet conversation oral or written.

* Walk 15 min.

* If you have invading thoughts about eating, ask yourself if it is possible to ignore them.

Yes

Great! In such a case continue ignoring them.

No

You have to learn to ignore the invading thoughts about eating.

This Guide will teach you to ignore the invading thoughts about eating.

Remember: even if you cannot stop the invading thoughts, the invading thoughts cannot stop you to live a normal life.

If you believe in things which other people consider strange, try to keep your strange believes for yourself. Everybody has to make the selection of what can be told to other people and what must be private. Believe me, many people have strange believes. Even much stranger than yours. And they are not considered to be

sick. Why? Because they keep their strange believes for themselves. That is the secret.

***

Afternoon

* Say slowly whenever you are invaded by the thoughts about eating: sun, flower, seven, path, tee, run, yellow, apple, fish, rain, pen, water, smile, talk, life, sky.

* Think of three different words, any words which just come to your mind at the moment and make a simple story using these 3 words. Repeat 3 times.

* Try to concentrate on an object close to you, any object. What do you feel when looking at the object? What thoughts come to your mind when looking at the object? And why?Maybe there is a reason. Look for the reason but not too long. If you don't find the reason, forget it.

* Dinner and half an hour break (you can sleep).

* Nice talk (no complaints) 15 min. When nobody to talk with, phone or internet conversation oral or written.

* Walk 20 min.

* If you have the invading thoughts about eating, ask yourself if it is possible to ignore them.

Yes

Great! In such a case continue ignoring them.

No

You have to learn to ignore the invading thoughts.

This Guide will teach you to ignore the invading thoughts about eating.

Remember: even if you cannot stop the invading thoughts, the invading thoughts cannot stop you to live a normal life.

If you believe in things which other people consider strange, try to keep your strange believes for yourself. Everybody has to make the selection of what can be told to other people and what must be private. Believe me, many people have strange believes. Even much stranger than yours. And they are not considered to be sick. Why? Because they keep their strange believes for themselves. That is the secret.

***

Evening

- Say slowly whenever you are invaded by the thoughts about eating: sun, flower, seven, path, tee, run, yellow, apple, fish, rain, pen, water, smile, talk, life, sky.

- Think of three different words, any words which just come to your mind at the moment and make a simple story using these 3 words. Repeat 3 times.
  - Try to concentrate on an object close to you, any object. What do you feel when looking at the object? What thoughts come to your mind when looking at the object? And why? Maybe there is a reason. Look for the reason but not too long. If you don't find the reason, forget it.
  - Small supper.
  - Nice talk (no complaints) 10 min. When nobody to talk with, phone or internet conversation oral or written.
  - Walk 10 min.
  - If you have the invading thoughts about eating, ask yourself if it is possible to ignore them.

Yes

Great! In such a case continue ignoring them.

No

You have to learn to ignore the invading thoughts.

This Guide will teach you to ignore the invading thoughts.

Remember: even if you cannot stop the invading thoughts, the invading thoughts cannot stop you to live a normal life.

If you believe in things which other people consider strange, try to keep your strange believes for yourself. Everybody has to make the selection of what can be told to other people and what must be private. Believe me, many people have strange believes. Even much stranger than yours. And they are not considered to be sick. Why? Because they keep their strange believes for themselves. That is the secret.

***

Night

Before sleep

- Take a shower (warm water) 1 min.
- Small physical excercise 3 min.

In Bed

- Repeat STOP (10 times if you have invading thoughts).

- Say slowly whenever you are invaded by the thoughts about eating: sun, flower, seven, path, tee, run, yellow, apple, fish, rain, pen, water, smile, talk, life, sky.
- Think of three different words, any words which just come to your mind at the moment and make a simple story using these 3 words. Repeat untill you fall asleep.

If you cannot fall asleep

- Say slowly whenever you are invaded by the thoughts about eating: sun, flower, seven, path, tee, run, yellow, apple, fish, rain, pen, water, smile, talk, life, sky.

If you cannot asleep

- Think of three different words, any words which just come to your mind at the moment and make a simple story using these 3 words. Repeat untill you fall asleep.

If above does not help

- Stand up and go to the toilet (when possible with as little light as possible)
- Say slowly whenever you are invaded by the thoughts about eating: sun, flower, seven, path,

tee, run, yellow, apple, fish, rain, pen, water, smile, talk, life, sky.
- Think of three different words, any words which just come to your mind at the moment and make a simple story using these 3 words. Repeat untill you fall asleep.

If above does not help

- Say STOP untill you fall asleep

If above does not help

- Go to the kitchen and have a very small snack.
- Back to the bed think of three different words, any words which just come to your mind at the moment and make a simple story using these 3 words. Repeat untill you fall asleep.
- If above does not help think of three different words, any words which just come to your mind at the moment and make a simple story using these 3 words. Repeat untill you fall asleep.
- Say slowly whenever you are invaded by the thoughts about eating: sun, flower, seven, path, tee, run, yellow, apple, fish, rain, pen, water, smile, talk, life, sky. Repeat untill you fall asleep.

***

Day 5

Morning

* Say STOP whenever thoughts about eating come to your mind.

* Say slowly whenever you are invaded by the thoughts about eating: sun, flower, seven, path, tee, run, yellow, apple, fish, rain, pen, water, smile, talk, life, sky.

* If above does not help to stop the thoughts about eating just turn your attention away from the invading thoughts about eating. The best way to turn your attention away from the invading thoughts about eating in your head is by doing one of your favorite occupations. Do not be ashamed of any occupation to turn your attention away from the invading thoughts in your head. ALWAYS be busy with your favorite occupation when unsupportable thoughts come to your head.

* Be careful to keep for yourself these of your believes which are found to be strange by the people.

* CONTROL what you say. Say only things which are not strange for the people. You surely already know which of your believes are found to be strange by the people.

* If you do not know yet which of your believes are found to be strange by the people, OBSERVE how

people react on what you say. If you see that people are ALERTED by your believes, it means your believes are strange. From now on AVOID presenting such believes.

* Think of three different words, any words which just come to your mind at the moment and make a simple story using these 3 words. Repeat 3 times.

* Try to concentrate on an object close to you, any object. What do you feel when looking at the object? What thoughts come to your mind when looking at the object? And why? Maybe there is a reason. Look for the reason but not too long. If you don't find the reason, forget it.

* Small physical excercise (10 min)

* Small breakfast.

* Nice talk (no complaints, no problematic questions) 10 min. When nobody to talk with, phone or internet conversation oral or written.

* Walk 15 min.

* If you have invading thoughts about eating, ask yourself if it is possible to ignore them.

Yes

Great! In such a case continue ignoring them.

No

You have to learn to ignore the invading thoughts about eating.

This Guide will teach you to ignore the invading thoughts about eating.

Remember: even if you cannot stop the invading thoughts, the invading thoughts cannot stop you to live a normal life.

If you believe in things which other people consider strange, try to keep your strange believes for yourself. Everybody has to make the selection of what can be told to other people and what must be private. Believe me, many people have strange believes. Even much stranger than yours. And they are not considered to be sick. Why? Because they keep their strange believes for themselves. That is the secret.

***

Afternoon

* Say slowly whenever you are invaded by the thoughts about eating: sun, flower, seven, path, tee, run, yellow, apple, fish, rain, pen, water, smile, talk, life, sky.

* Think of three different words, any words which just come to your mind at the moment and make a simple story using these 3 words. Repeat 3 times.

* Try to concentrate on an object close to you, any object. What do you feel when looking at the object? What thoughts come to your mind when looking at the object? And why?Maybe there is a reason. Look for the reason but not too long. If you don't find the reason, forget it.

* Dinner and half an hour break (you can sleep).

* Nice talk (no complaints) 15 min. When nobody to talk with, phone or internet conversation oral or written.

* Walk 20 min.

* If you have the invading thoughts about eating, ask yourself if it is possible to ignore them.

Yes

Great! In such a case continue ignoring them.

No

You have to learn to ignore the invading thoughts.

This Guide will teach you to ignore the invading thoughts about eating.

Remember: even if you cannot stop the invading thoughts, the invading thoughts cannot stop you to live a normal life.

If you believe in things which other people consider strange, try to keep your strange believes for yourself. Everybody has to make the selection of what can be told to other people and what must be private. Believe me, many people have strange believes. Even much stranger than yours. And they are not considered to be sick. Why? Because they keep their strange believes for themselves. That is the secret.

***

Evening

- Say slowly whenever you are invaded by the thoughts about eating: sun, flower, seven, path, tee, run, yellow, apple, fish, rain, pen, water, smile, talk, life, sky.

- Think of three different words, any words which just come to your mind at the moment and make a simple story using these 3 words. Repeat 3 times.
  - Try to concentrate on an object close to you, any object. What do you feel when looking at the object? What thoughts come to your mind when

looking at the object? And why? Maybe there is a reason. Look for the reason but not too long. If you don't find the reason, forget it.
- Small supper.
- Nice talk (no complaints) 10 min. When nobody to talk with, phone or internet conversation oral or written.
- Walk 10 min.
- If you have the invading thoughts about eating, ask yourself if it is possible to ignore them.

Yes

Great! In such a case continue ignoring them.

No

You have to learn to ignore the invading thoughts.

This Guide will teach you to ignore the invading thoughts.

Remember: even if you cannot stop the invading thoughts, the invading thoughts cannot stop you to live a normal life.

If you believe in things which other people consider strange, try to keep your strange believes for yourself. Everybody has to make the selection of what can be told to other people and what must be private. Believe

me, many people have strange believes. Even much stranger than yours. And they are not considered to be sick. Why? Because they keep their strange believes for themselves. That is the secret.

***

Night

Before sleep

- Take a shower (warm water) 1 min.
- Small physical excercise 3 min.

In Bed

- Repeat STOP (10 times if you have invading thoughts).
- Say slowly whenever you are invaded by the thoughts about eating: sun, flower, seven, path, tee, run, yellow, apple, fish, rain, pen, water, smile, talk, life, sky.
- Think of three different words, any words which just come to your mind at the moment and make a simple story using these 3 words. Repeat untill you fall asleep.

If you cannot fall asleep

- Say slowly whenever you are invaded by the thoughts about eating: sun, flower, seven, path,

tee, run, yellow, apple, fish, rain, pen, water, smile, talk, life, sky.

If you cannot asleep

- Think of three different words, any words which just come to your mind at the moment and make a simple story using these 3 words. Repeat untill you fall asleep.

If above does not help

- Stand up and go to the toilet (when possible with as little light as possible)
- Say slowly whenever you are invaded by the thoughts about eating: sun, flower, seven, path, tee, run, yellow, apple, fish, rain, pen, water, smile, talk, life, sky.
- Think of three different words, any words which just come to your mind at the moment and make a simple story using these 3 words. Repeat untill you fall asleep.

If above does not help

- Say STOP untill you fall asleep

If above does not help

- Go to the kitchen and have a very small snack.

- Back to the bed think of three different words, any words which just come to your mind at the moment and make a simple story using these 3 words. Repeat untill you fall asleep.
- If above does not help think of three different words, any words which just come to your mind at the moment and make a simple story using these 3 words. Repeat untill you fall asleep.
- Say slowly whenever you are invaded by the thoughts about eating: sun, flower, seven, path, tee, run, yellow, apple, fish, rain, pen, water, smile, talk, life, sky. Repeat untill you fall asleep.

***

Day 6

Morning

* Say STOP whenever thoughts about eating come to your mind.

* Say slowly whenever you are invaded by the thoughts about eating: sun, flower, seven, path, tee, run, yellow, apple, fish, rain, pen, water, smile, talk, life, sky.

* If above does not help to stop the thoughts about eating just turn your attention away from the invading thoughts about eating. The best way to turn your

attention away from the invading thoughts about eating in your head is by doing one of your favorite occupations. Do not be ashamed of any occupation to turn your attention away from the invading thoughts in your head. ALWAYS be busy with your favorite occupation when unsupportable thoughts come to your head.

* Be careful to keep for yourself these of your believes which are found to be strange by the people.

* CONTROL what you say. Say only things which are not strange for the people. You surely already know which of your believes are found to be strange by the people.

* If you do not know yet which of your believes are found to be strange by the people, OBSERVE how people react on what you say. If you see that people are ALERTED by your believes, it means your believes are strange. From now on AVOID presenting such believes.

* Think of three different words, any words which just come to your mind at the moment and make a simple story using these 3 words. Repeat 3 times.

* Try to concentrate on an object close to you, any object. What do you feel when looking at the object? What thoughts come to your mind when looking at the object? And why? Maybe there is a reason. Look for the

reason but not too long. If you don't find the reason, forget it.

* Small physical excercise (10 min)

* Small breakfast.

* Nice talk (no complaints, no problematic questions) 10 min. When nobody to talk with, phone or internet conversation oral or written.

* Walk 15 min.

* If you have invading thoughts about eating, ask yourself if it is possible to ignore them.

Yes

Great! In such a case continue ignoring them.

No

You have to learn to ignore the invading thoughts about eating.

This Guide will teach you to ignore the invading thoughts about eating.

Remember: even if you cannot stop the invading thoughts, the invading thoughts cannot stop you to live a normal life.

If you believe in things which other people consider strange, try to keep your strange believes for yourself. Everybody has to make the selection of what can be told to other people and what must be private. Believe me, many people have strange believes. Even much stranger than yours. And they are not considered to be sick. Why? Because they keep their strange believes for themselves. That is the secret.

***

Afternoon

* Say slowly whenever you are invaded by the thoughts about eating: sun, flower, seven, path, tee, run, yellow, apple, fish, rain, pen, water, smile, talk, life, sky.

* Think of three different words, any words which just come to your mind at the moment and make a simple story using these 3 words. Repeat 3 times.

* Try to concentrate on an object close to you, any object. What do you feel when looking at the object? What thoughts come to your mind when looking at the object? And why?Maybe there is a reason. Look for the reason but not too long. If you don't find the reason, forget it.

* Dinner and half an hour break (you can sleep).

* Nice talk (no complaints) 15 min. When nobody to talk with, phone or internet conversation oral or written.

* Walk 20 min.

* If you have the invading thoughts about eating, ask yourself if it is possible to ignore them.

Yes

Great! In such a case continue ignoring them.

No

You have to learn to ignore the invading thoughts.

This Guide will teach you to ignore the invading thoughts about eating.

Remember: even if you cannot stop the invading thoughts, the invading thoughts cannot stop you to live a normal life.

If you believe in things which other people consider strange, try to keep your strange believes for yourself. Everybody has to make the selection of what can be told to other people and what must be private. Believe me, many people have strange believes. Even much stranger than yours. And they are not considered to be

sick. Why? Because they keep their strange believes for themselves. That is the secret.

***

Evening

- Say slowly whenever you are invaded by the thoughts about eating: sun, flower, seven, path, tee, run, yellow, apple, fish, rain, pen, water, smile, talk, life, sky.

- Think of three different words, any words which just come to your mind at the moment and make a simple story using these 3 words. Repeat 3 times.
  - Try to concentrate on an object close to you, any object. What do you feel when looking at the object? What thoughts come to your mind when looking at the object? And why? Maybe there is a reason. Look for the reason but not too long. If you don't find the reason, forget it.
  - Small supper.
  - Nice talk (no complaints) 10 min. When nobody to talk with, phone or internet conversation oral or written.
  - Walk 10 min.
  - If you have the invading thoughts about eating, ask yourself if it is possible to ignore them.

Yes

Great! In such a case continue ignoring them.

No

You have to learn to ignore the invading thoughts.

This Guide will teach you to ignore the invading thoughts.

Remember: even if you cannot stop the invading thoughts, the invading thoughts cannot stop you to live a normal life.

If you believe in things which other people consider strange, try to keep your strange believes for yourself. Everybody has to make the selection of what can be told to other people and what must be private. Believe me, many people have strange believes. Even much stranger than yours. And they are not considered to be sick. Why? Because they keep their strange believes for themselves. That is the secret.

***

Night

Before sleep

- Take a shower (warm water) 1 min.
- Small physical excercise 3 min.

In Bed

- Repeat STOP (10 times if you have invading thoughts).
- Say slowly whenever you are invaded by the thoughts about eating: sun, flower, seven, path, tee, run, yellow, apple, fish, rain, pen, water, smile, talk, life, sky.
- Think of three different words, any words which just come to your mind at the moment and make a simple story using these 3 words. Repeat untill you fall asleep.

If you cannot fall asleep

- Say slowly whenever you are invaded by the thoughts about eating: sun, flower, seven, path, tee, run, yellow, apple, fish, rain, pen, water, smile, talk, life, sky.

If you cannot asleep

- Think of three different words, any words which just come to your mind at the moment and make a simple story using these 3 words. Repeat untill you fall asleep.

If above does not help

- Stand up and go to the toilet (when possible with as little light as possible)

- Say slowly whenever you are invaded by the thoughts about eating: sun, flower, seven, path, tee, run, yellow, apple, fish, rain, pen, water, smile, talk, life, sky.
- Think of three different words, any words which just come to your mind at the moment and make a simple story using these 3 words. Repeat untill you fall asleep.

If above does not help

- Say STOP untill you fall asleep

If above does not help

- Go to the kitchen and have a very small snack.
- Back to the bed think of three different words, any words which just come to your mind at the moment and make a simple story using these 3 words. Repeat untill you fall asleep.
- If above does not help think of three different words, any words which just come to your mind at the moment and make a simple story using these 3 words. Repeat untill you fall asleep.
- Say slowly whenever you are invaded by the thoughts about eating: sun, flower, seven, path, tee, run, yellow, apple, fish, rain, pen, water, smile, talk, life, sky. Repeat untill you fall asleep.

***

Day 7

Morning

* Say STOP whenever thoughts about eating come to your mind.

* Say slowly whenever you are invaded by the thoughts about eating: sun, flower, seven, path, tee, run, yellow, apple, fish, rain, pen, water, smile, talk, life, sky.

* If above does not help to stop the thoughts about eating just turn your attention away from the invading thoughts about eating. The best way to turn your attention away from the invading thoughts about eating in your head is by doing one of your favorite occupations. Do not be ashamed of any occupation to turn your attention away from the invading thoughts in your head. ALWAYS be busy with your favorite occupation when unsupportable thoughts come to your head.

* Be careful to keep for yourself these of your believes which are found to be strange by the people.

* CONTROL what you say. Say only things which are not strange for the people. You surely already know which of your believes are found to be strange by the people.

* If you do not know yet which of your believes are found to be strange by the people, OBSERVE how people react on what you say. If you see that people are ALERTED by your believes, it means your believes are strange. From now on AVOID presenting such believes.

* Think of three different words, any words which just come to your mind at the moment and make a simple story using these 3 words. Repeat 3 times.

* Try to concentrate on an object close to you, any object. What do you feel when looking at the object? What thoughts come to your mind when looking at the object? And why? Maybe there is a reason. Look for the reason but not too long. If you don't find the reason, forget it.

* Small physical excercise (10 min)

* Small breakfast.

* Nice talk (no complaints, no problematic questions) 10 min. When nobody to talk with, phone or internet conversation oral or written.

* Walk 15 min.

* If you have invading thoughts about eating, ask yourself if it is possible to ignore them.

Yes

Great! In such a case continue ignoring them.

No

You have to learn to ignore the invading thoughts about eating.

This Guide will teach you to ignore the invading thoughts about eating.

Remember: even if you cannot stop the invading thoughts, the invading thoughts cannot stop you to live a normal life.

If you believe in things which other people consider strange, try to keep your strange believes for yourself. Everybody has to make the selection of what can be told to other people and what must be private. Believe me, many people have strange believes. Even much stranger than yours. And they are not considered to be sick. Why? Because they keep their strange believes for themselves. That is the secret.

***

Afternoon

* Say slowly whenever you are invaded by the thoughts about eating: sun, flower, seven, path, tee, run, yellow, apple, fish, rain, pen, water, smile, talk, life, sky.

* Think of three different words, any words which just come to your mind at the moment and make a simple story using these 3 words. Repeat 3 times.

* Try to concentrate on an object close to you, any object. What do you feel when looking at the object? What thoughts come to your mind when looking at the object? And why? Maybe there is a reason. Look for the reason but not too long. If you don't find the reason, forget it.

* Dinner and half an hour break (you can sleep).

* Nice talk (no complaints) 15 min. When nobody to talk with, phone or internet conversation oral or written.

* Walk 20 min.

* If you have the invading thoughts about eating, ask yourself if it is possible to ignore them.

Yes

Great! In such a case continue ignoring them.

No

You have to learn to ignore the invading thoughts.

This Guide will teach you to ignore the invading thoughts about eating.

Remember: even if you cannot stop the invading thoughts, the invading thoughts cannot stop you to live a normal life.

If you believe in things which other people consider strange, try to keep your strange believes for yourself. Everybody has to make the selection of what can be told to other people and what must be private. Believe me, many people have strange believes. Even much stranger than yours. And they are not considered to be sick. Why? Because they keep their strange believes for themselves. That is the secret.

***

Evening

- Say slowly whenever you are invaded by the thoughts about eating: sun, flower, seven, path, tee, run, yellow, apple, fish, rain, pen, water, smile, talk, life, sky.

- Think of three different words, any words which just come to your mind at the moment and make a simple story using these 3 words. Repeat 3 times.

- Try to concentrate on an object close to you, any object. What do you feel when looking at the object? What thoughts come to your mind when looking at the object? And why? Maybe there is a reason. Look for the reason but not too long. If you don't find the reason, forget it.
- Small supper.
- Nice talk (no complaints) 10 min. When nobody to talk with, phone or internet conversation oral or written.
- Walk 10 min.
- If you have the invading thoughts about eating, ask yourself if it is possible to ignore them.

Yes

Great! In such a case continue ignoring them.

No

You have to learn to ignore the invading thoughts.

This Guide will teach you to ignore the invading thoughts.

Remember: even if you cannot stop the invading thoughts, the invading thoughts cannot stop you to live a normal life.

If you believe in things which other people consider strange, try to keep your strange believes for yourself. Everybody has to make the selection of what can be told to other people and what must be private. Believe me, many people have strange believes. Even much stranger than yours. And they are not considered to be sick. Why? Because they keep their strange believes for themselves. That is the secret.

***

Night

Before sleep

- Take a shower (warm water) 1 min.
- Small physical excercise 3 min.

In Bed

- Repeat STOP (10 times if you have invading thoughts).
- Say slowly whenever you are invaded by the thoughts about eating: sun, flower, seven, path, tee, run, yellow, apple, fish, rain, pen, water, smile, talk, life, sky.
- Think of three different words, any words which just come to your mind at the moment and make a simple story using these 3 words. Repeat untill you fall asleep.

If you cannot fall asleep

- Say slowly whenever you are invaded by the thoughts about eating: sun, flower, seven, path, tee, run, yellow, apple, fish, rain, pen, water, smile, talk, life, sky.

If you cannot asleep

- Think of three different words, any words which just come to your mind at the moment and make a simple story using these 3 words. Repeat untill you fall asleep.

If above does not help

- Stand up and go to the toilet (when possible with as little light as possible)
- Say slowly whenever you are invaded by the thoughts about eating: sun, flower, seven, path, tee, run, yellow, apple, fish, rain, pen, water, smile, talk, life, sky.
- Think of three different words, any words which just come to your mind at the moment and make a simple story using these 3 words. Repeat untill you fall asleep.

If above does not help

- Say STOP untill you fall asleep

If above does not help

- Go to the kitchen and have a very small snack.
- Back to the bed think of three different words, any words which just come to your mind at the moment and make a simple story using these 3 words. Repeat untill you fall asleep.
- If above does not help think of three different words, any words which just come to your mind at the moment and make a simple story using these 3 words. Repeat untill you fall asleep.
- Say slowly whenever you are invaded by the thoughts about eating: sun, flower, seven, path, tee, run, yellow, apple, fish, rain, pen, water, smile, talk, life, sky. Repeat untill you fall asleep.

***

Congratulations! You made the Eating Disorder Self Therapy! Now you have the invading thoughts about eating under control and you are ready to live a full and happy life. Good luck!!! And come back to this Guide whenever the invading thoughts about eating reappear.

P. W. Ariveder

www.ingramcontent.com/pod-product-compliance
Lightning Source LLC
Chambersburg PA
CBHW052340220526
45465CB00003BA/886